HYSTERECTOMY

WANDA WIGFALL-WILLIAMS

Hysterectomy

LEARNING THE FACTS

COPING WITH THE FEELINGS

FACING THE FUTURE

Michael Kesend Publishing, Ltd. · New York

Library of Congress Cataloging-in-Publication Data

Wigfall-Williams, Wanda, 1953-
    Hysterectomy: learning the facts, coping with the feelings, facing the future.
    Bibliography: p.
    Includes index.
    1. Hysterectomy—Popular Works,   I. Title
[DNLM: 1. Hysterectomy—popular works. WP 468 W654h]
RG391.W54   1986   618.1'453   86-7317
ISBN 0-935576-15-0 (paper)
ISBN 0-935576-17-7 (cloth)

This book does not intend to treat, diagnose, or prescribe and therefore does not take responsibility for your experience using information contained therein.

Book design: Jackie Schuman
Illustrations: Maryann Ginsberg

For David, Chris and Lucy,
whose love, support and encouragement
helped make this book possible.

C O N T E N T S

ACKNOWLEDGMENTS

This book is a combination of many efforts. I am thankful to Dr. Edmund Petrilli, Dr. Richard Edelson, Dr. Michael Shefferman and Dr. Lucy Waletzky for their help in reviewing the medical sections of this book.

My editor, Jane Pincus, has helped through the many improvements she has suggested. I am grateful for the endorsement that Gail Ross of Goldfarb & Singer gave to the book when she agreed to represent me, and to Michael Kesend for deciding to publish it. Nancy Shands, Joan Lindsey, Karen Timmons and Kate Weinstein have helped by contributing ideas and suggestions to this project.

In addition, the book was enriched by the women and men who allowed me to interview them about deeply personal experiences.

HYSTERECTOMY

PROLOGUE

Nearly three-quarters of a million American women will undergo hyster-ectomy this year. Approximately 30 percent of those hysterectomies will be performed unnecessarily. Most women will be ill-prepared for the physical and psychological trauma. If you must deal with this surgery, you'll feel more comfortable if you arm yourself with knowledge about the choices you'll be forced to face before, during and after.

While the overall numbers of hysterectomies have been decreasing, the number of hysterectomies performed on women in the fifteen to forty-four age group has increased markedly. According to the Center for Disease Control (CDC) and Washington, D.C., gynecologists, the reason for this increase is earlier detection of benign (noncancerous) gynecologic diseases—endometriosis, fibroids, adenomyosis and pelvic inflammatory disease (PID)—and cancer. It is not that more women have such conditions but that new diagnostic techniques enable doctors to identify them sooner than they could in the past. These diseases are usually first discovered when a woman has trouble becoming pregnant.

In the following pages I discuss the medical conditions which can bring a woman face to face with hysterectomy. This book provides step-by-step guidance through the maze of decisions and problems precipi-tated by the prospect of hysterectomy. Designed to help demystify the entire experience, it offers suggestions, tools and vital information designed to make your hysterectomy more manageable and tolerable.

This book is also geared toward helping you take the best possible care of yourself. Make absolutely certain that the operation is necessary.

I advise this because doctors have performed many unnecessary hysterectomies and oophorectomies (removal of ovaries). In the case of older women, they judged that reproductive organs were no longer necessary for childbearing and at potential risk for cancer, and so removed the uterus and ovaries. Some also used hysterectomy as first choice of treatment for minor problems including mood swings and premenstrual syndrome. In fact, the hysterectomy rate has leveled off, in great part because both women and doctors have become more knowledgeable about more conservative methods of treatment for minor conditions. Ironically, in some larger cities, a new trend seems to be developing: some women are having difficulty in getting *necessary* hysterectomies. This might be happening because doctors want to try other treatment methods, or because they fear malpractice suits.

Since the majority of hysterectomies (90–95 percent) are performed on an elective (nonemergency) basis, most women will be able to follow the guidelines described in this book to help determine whether or not hysterectomy is the best choice. However, if you are in a crisis situation and do not have time to make inquiries regarding physicians and your disease, your only recourse will be to learn as much as you can on the spot. This book can help you deal with the aftermath.

Women facing hysterectomy are often frightened by the experience because they lack useful information. I hope to address your most common fears and allay most anxieties with comprehensive, intelligent information regarding the physical, emotional and sexual ramifications of this experience, giving you appropriate tools for dealing with the surgery and emerging from it in good health emotionally and physically.

Why Hysterectomy May Be Necessary

Last year, approximately 700,000 hysterectomies were performed on women in the United States. According to the most recent statistics,[1] there has been a 57 percent overall increase since 1965 and a 71 percent increase in the number of women in the fifteen to forty-four age range. Once thought of as a prophylactic surgery to be performed on postmenopausal women, hysterectomy is fast becoming a fact of life—a rather painful fact (physiologically, psychologically, and sexually)—for a larger and younger segment of the female population.

Except in advanced cases of cancer, or in a crisis situation (such as hemorrhaging), you should consider hysterectomy only after more conservative treatment methods have been tried and found to be ineffective.

COMMON DISORDERS FOR WHICH HYSTERECTOMY MAY BE NECESSARY

The most common diseases for which hysterectomy is considered the best treatment when all else fails are:

Fibroids (see figure 1.1). This is one of the most common conditions for which hysterectomy is advised. Fibroids (*leiomyoma* in medical terminology) refer to common uterine growths composed of connective tissue and muscle fiber which originate from the muscle wall of the uterus. Almost all diagnosed cases of fibroid tumors are benign (non-cancerous). Rarely does a benign fibroid become malignant. There are,

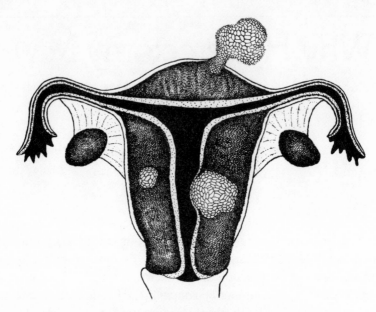

Figure 1.1   Fibroids

Fibroids (leiomyoma in medical terminology) refer to the common uterine growths composed of connective tissue and muscle fiber originating from the muscle wall of the uterus. Shown here are: intramural fibroids which are located deep inside the uterine wall and when they grow these fibroids may block the fallopian tubes; submucosal fibroids which extend from the uterine lining into the uterus causing bleeding; and subserous fibroids which grow outside of the uterus causing problems as they become large and twist.

however, less common cases in which the fibroids are malignant (cancerous). In this situation, the fibroid will grow quite rapidly and the change in size will be detectable through a pelvic examination and other diagnostic tests such as ultrasonography. Fibroid tumors appear to be estrogen dependent. It is during childbearing years that estrogen levels are at their highest. This is when women are at the greatest risk. Premenstruating women and postmenopausal women are seldom plagued by this condition. There are several types of fibroids:

> *subserous fibroids* protrude from the surface of the pelvic cavity into the uterus
> *intramural fibroids* are located deep inside the uterine wall

submucosal fibroids extend from the endometrial lining into the uterine cavity

Before considering hysterectomy, it would be useful to pursue a more conservative treatment approach. You can ask several questions to help determine the best course of treatment.

1. How large are the fibroids? If they are very small and cause little or no discomfort, the doctor may suggest that no treatment be started. He/she may decide to monitor the fibroids' growth on a regular checkup schedule.
2. Are the fibroids causing abnormal bleeding? If they are small, but cause abnormal bleeding, the doctor may want to start hormone therapy (usually progesterone) to help stop the bleeding, and schedule regular office visits to monitor the fibroids' growth.
3. Assuming that diagnostic tests rule out cancer, is it possible to wait out the fibroid symptoms (irregular bleeding and pain) until menopause? Postmenopausal women do not usually have problems with fibroids.

If it is not possible to manage the problem with noninvasive methods, a myomectomy (a procedure in which the fibroid is removed but the uterus is left in place) should be the first surgical consideration for this condition. A hysterectomy might be necessary if any of these conditions is present: uncontrolled bleeding, extremely large fibroids (large usually refers to a fibroid equivalent in size to a twelve-week fetus, approximately 7cm in length), or if malignancy is suspected.

Endometriosis (see figure 1.2). This is a condition in which endometrial tissue (lining of the uterus) begins growing in various sites outside the uterus. These growths, referred to as implants, commonly attach themselves to the ovaries, fallopian tubes, bladder, and rectum as well as other parts of the abdominal cavity. These implants function as though they continue to be part of the uterine lining, in that they thicken and bleed into the pelvic cavity each month in accordance with the ovarian cycle. These implants, which are almost always benign, may grow between two organs, forming adhesions (see figure 1.2). Because

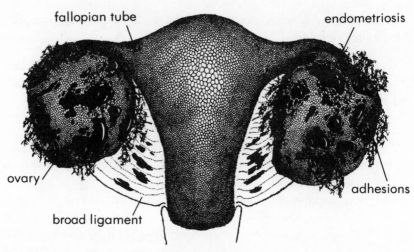

Figure 1.2   Endometriosis
Endometriotic Implants, or "chocolate cysts," are shown attached to the
ovaries, fallopian tubes, and broad ligaments. In addition, hemorrhagic shaggy
tissue, also known as adhesions, is often found in women with endometriosis.

of the adhesions and scarring caused by endometriosis, women are
often in great pain.

Endometriosis is usually confirmed by a laparoscopy, a procedure in
which the physician inserts a narrow tube into the pelvic cavity through
a small incision in the navel. The physician can then look at the ovaries
and tubes and make a positive identification of the disease. Laparoscopy has its limitations because the doctor cannot see the entire pelvic
cavity. Therefore, a woman might have endometriosis in an area not
visible to the doctor. If the disease is serious enough to warrant medical
attention, the first course of action is a noninvasive approach (nonsurgi-
cal). Hormonal therapy is usually the first course the doctor will pursue.
Danazol is the leading drug used currently although others (Provera and
low dose birth control pills) may be more appropriate for you. Your
physician will start treating you with a drug that offers the least number
of side effects given your medical history. Women who can't tolerate
Danazol often respond successfully to low dose birth control pills and/or
progesterone. Because hormonal therapy may be ineffective against
endometriosis, surgery (laser or conventional) to remove the implants

may be recommended. Laser surgery involves using an intense beam of light to remove endometriosis and scar tissue. Many doctors prefer this type of surgery because blood loss is minimal and the recuperation period shorter. Laser surgery is sometimes used in conjunction with conventional surgery (using a scalpel to remove the implants) to treat endometriosis. If a woman is considering having children or is very young, this option may be very appealing. However, because endometriosis is estrogen dependent, as long as the ovaries remain functional, new sites of endometriosis may arise. If a woman has tried all forms of conservative treatments and is still suffering from the disease, hysterectomy with oophorectomy may be the best alternative.

Adenomyosis (see figure 1.3). This condition is most commonly seen in women in their forties, usually after the peak of their childbearing years. The endometrial tissue penetrates the uterine wall and makes it thick, spongy and tender. Abdominal pain and prolonged periods with heavy bleeding are the most common symptoms. Some gynecologists take a noninvasive approach to treatment initially by prescribing Dana-

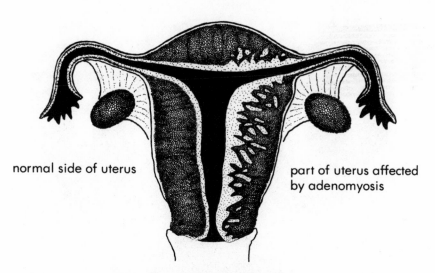

normal side of uterus

part of uterus affected by adenomyosis

Figure 1.3 Adenomyosis
This figure is a cross section of a uterus. The left side is normal, while the right side of the uterus is affected by the disease.

zol (same drug often used in treatment of endometriosis) or Provera (another hormone) in combination with an antiprostaglandin (which blocks the normal activity of hormones) such as Motrin, Ponstel or Anaprox. If this form of treatment is not effective, then hysterectomy may be the only other alternative.[2] Diagnosis of adenomyosis is very difficult. There are, however, some symptoms that may indicate such a disorder:

> *Enlarged uterus*—the uterus will become larger, but usually larger symmetrically.
> *Age of patient*—this disorder occurs most frequently in older women.
> *Pelvic pain*—pelvic pain is the major complaint with adenomyosis.
> *Bladder or bowel irritation*—the bladder and bowel are tender and show some signs of abnormal functioning.

If the lesion is localized, an attempt will be made to resect (cut out the diseased portion of) the uterine wall. However, because adenomyosis usually spreads throughout the uterine muscle wall, hysterectomy is the

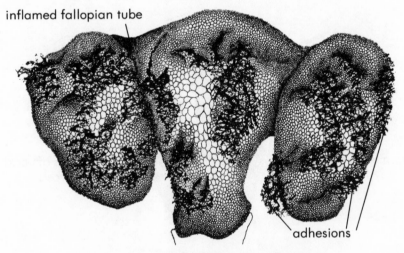

Figure 1.4   Pelvic Inflammatory Disease
This figure illustrates what happens in the pelvic cavity as a result of Pelvic Inflammatory Disease. The ovaries, fallopian tubes and uterus become inflamed and often scarring and adhesions are formed.

more complete course of treatment. Absolute diagnosis of adenomyosis can be confirmed only after the uterus has been removed and the tissue examined by a pathologist.

Pelvic Inflammatory Disease (see figure 1.4). Pelvic Inflammatory Disease (PID) is a catch-all term encompassing all sexually transmitted diseases (STDs) that impact on the gynecological health of a woman. PID may be caused by one of several bacterial infections, including but not limited to chlamydia and gonococcus. Directly or indirectly involved in approximately 20 percent of all gynecologic problems,[3] PID is an infectious process that may involve the ovaries, fallopian tubes, pelvic peritoneum (lining of the pelvis), veins or pelvic connective tissue. The infection may be confined to one structure, or may involve the entire pelvis. Pain is the most common symptom. The pain may be character-ized as dull cramping of intermittent frequency; or may be severe, sharp, persistent and incapacitating. The primary course of treatment is intensive, aggressive antibiotic therapy over a period of time. When the infection is so extensive that it does not respond to this type of treatment, hysterectomy may become necessary.

Cancer (see figure 1.5). Cancer refers to a group of diseases in which there is irregular growth of abnormal cells. While normal cells are of uniform size and shape and grow only to replace old cells, abnormal cells vary in size and shape, grow in an uncontrolled pattern and never stop producing. Eventually the malignant cells outnumber the healthy cells. Three main reproductive organs, when determined malignant, may require some form of hysterectomy as a life-saving form of treatment. The organs most frequently affected and the accompanying symptoms are:

CERVIX—There is only one type of cervical cancer. A precancerous condition, cervical cancer in situ, is one in which atypical cells are confined to the cervix. Excising the cervix through conization is the usual method of handling this disease. Forty-five years is the average age for *invasive cervical cancer.*[4] However, it is becoming increasingly common in younger women. The Pap smear, a diagnostic tool which involves analyzing a sample of cervical tissue, can be used to monitor

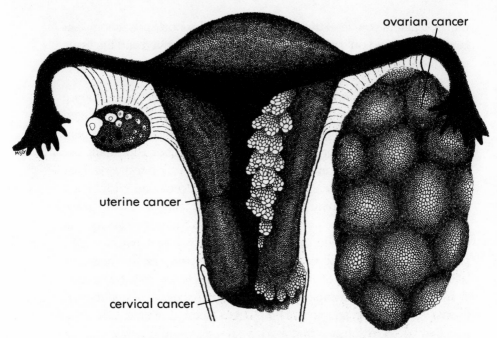

ovarian cancer

uterine cancer

cervical cancer

Figure 1.5   Reproductive System Malignancies

This figure illustrates malignancies of the ovary, uterus and cervix. The left side of the illustration is representative of the normal organ, while the right side illustrates its diseased state.

the status of a cervix that has atypical cells. Some characteristics of younger women who may be at risk are: low socioeconomic status, intercourse at an early age, early marriage, early age at first pregnancy, multiple pregnancies and inadequate care following delivery, multiple sex partners and exposure to venereal disease,[5] exposure to synthetic hormones (DES), and exposure to carcinogens in the workplace.

One of the earliest signs of invasive cervical cancer is abnormal bleeding and discharge. As the malignancy becomes larger, the bleeding becomes heavier and more frequent. A Pap smear is 80-85 percent accurate in diagnosing cervical cancer. It is possible to remove only the malignant tissue and leave the uterus, tubes and ovaries in place. However, this method does not guarantee a cure, and there is a chance that cancer may recur.

OVARIES—Ovarian cancer is fifth among the leading causes of cancer death in women.[6] Women at risk for this type of cancer are usually between the ages of forty and sixty years and the average age at the time of diagnosis is fifty-two years. Women most at risk have had a history of breast cancer, occupational exposure to asbestos, familial history of ovarian cancer, no history of pregnancy or first pregnancy after the age of thirty-five.

The most common symptoms of ovarian cancer are abnormal bleeding, pain, abdominal swelling, gastrointestinal distress (nausea, vomiting, diarrhea) and weight loss. The doctor usually discovers the enlarged ovary during the pelvic exam. A sonogram (a diagnostic tool which uses ultrasound waves rather than X rays to create an image) may be ordered to determine the size of the mass. Treatment for ovarian cancer is usually hysterectomy and bilateral salpingo-oophorectomy (removal of both fallopian tubes and ovaries). Conservative treatment, unilateral salpingo-oophorectomy (removal of one fallopian tube and ovary) may be done in order to preserve childbearing capability in younger women, provided the tumor is a low-grade malignancy[7] and confined to one ovary. Radiation and chemotherapy are often used as an adjunct treatment following surgery.

UTERUS—Uterine or endometrial cancer refers to a malignancy in the lining of the uterus. Postmenopausal women (women no longer menstruating) in the fifty to seventy age group are most at risk. Other risk factors include a history of abnormal bleeding, infertility, an ovarian malfunction, estrogen stimulation. (Often estrogen is prescribed by itself to control hot flashes, osteoporosis, vaginal atrophy, etc. However, more physicians are prescribing progesterone, a drug that balances the cell multiplying effect of estrogen, to counter the suspected negative effects of estrogen.) Abnormal uterine bleeding, abdominal and low back pain are the most common symptoms of uterine cancer. An enlarged uterus is often a sign of advanced uterine cancer. Uterine cancer is usually diagnosed through an endometrial biopsy or through a D&C (dilatation and curettage—this involves dilating the cervix and scraping out the uterine contents for examination). The most effective treatment is total abdominal hysterectomy with the removal of both ovaries and fallopian tubes (bilateral salpingo-oophorectomy), followed by radiation and/or hormonal therapy.

HOW TO RESEARCH YOUR DISEASE
AND ITS TREATMENTS

Learning from your physician that you have a condition for which hysterectomy is the best method of treatment is but the first bit of information necessary to make a responsible decision. It is your right and responsibility to be properly educated about your disease and the options for treatment. This goal may be achieved in the following ways:

INFORM YOURSELF

Consume all information concerning your condition. Medical school libraries, hospital libraries, consumer research groups such as Planetree Resource Center, The Boston Women's Health Book Collective (see Appendix 2 for addresses and description of services) and Medline (the on-line medical information service) are all excellent resources for reviewing past as well as current methods of treatment.

Most large hospital centers and medical colleges have access to Medline. You do not need special skills to get information regarding your disease. It is important to know the name of the disease and/or disorder and the particular type of information you'd like to get (newest surgical techniques, current medications used, and so forth). The librarian will take your request and program the computer to search for all the information that applies to your request. The cost for such a search can be anywhere from $40 to $100 depending on the amount of computer time used. For a listing of National Library of Medicine Regional Centers (centers in addition to medical colleges that have access to Medline), please see Appendix 2. For women living in large metropolitan areas obtaining medical information will be relatively easy. Women who live in rural areas and are unable to make the trip to a large city can arrange a search through one of the National Library of Medicine's Regional Center's librarians over the phone. Planetree Resource Center also handles phone requests for a wide range of subjects. Information about conservative and radical approaches as well as the benefits and liabilities is available. You don't have to be a doctor to fully understand the medical jargon, but a dictionary of medical terminology and an aggressive commitment to finding information are crucial.

Unless medical libraries and medical jargon are familiar territory, you should prepare yourself accordingly:

- Write down the exact name of the disease your doctor diagnosed.
- Write down the suggested treatment method.
- Go to the medical library and check the card file. If you have difficulty finding the information, ask the reference librarian. The reference staff will be more likely to assist you if you conduct your search during the day when most medical students are in class and the library staff has more time.
- Review the Medical Abstracts to get a list of current articles written on the subject. (There is a list of medical journals that address gynecological health in Appendix 2 that may be useful in gathering current information.)
- Make copies of pertinent articles, or make a list of questions to discuss with your physician. If alternative methods are discussed in the literature, be sure to make a copy of the treatment to give to your doctor so that he/she can go over it with you.
- Develop a list of questions and apprehensions and go over it carefully with your doctor (see sample questions for ideas).

ASK QUESTIONS

The questions here are ones that might be asked by a woman suffering with severe endometriosis. You can formulate other questions to address your specific needs.

1. Since I am not responding to Danazol, is there another drug that I could try before having surgery?
2. How many times can surgery be safely performed to remove endometriosis implants?
3. What type of hysterectomy are you going to perform?
4. Will it be possible for me to keep my ovaries and tubes?
5. If you have to remove my ovaries, will I experience menopausal symptoms after surgery?
6. Will a hysterectomy cure me?
7. What sort of incision will you have to make?

8. How long will this procedure take?
9. Will this surgery have any effect on me sexually?
10. How long will it be necessary to be hospitalized?
11. When will I be able to return to work?
12. When will I be able to begin an exercise program?
13. If you do remove my ovaries, will I need to start on hormonal replacement therapy immediately after surgery?
14. When will I get the pathologist's results?

GET A SECOND OPINION
Now that you have gathered the pertinent information and discussed with your physician all of your questions and fears, it is time to seek a second opinion.

Some women are reluctant to seek a second opinion out of fear of hurting their attending physician's feelings. Most physicians understand the importance of a second opinion to their patients and are willing to cooperate with you in terms of providing diagnostic test results and other useful information to the second opinion physician. When seeking a second opinion be certain to select a physician who is not in any way affiliated with the first doctor, and preferably a physician who operates at a different hospital from the first. By taking these precautions you are better able to assure an objective second opinion. Insurance companies, in their attempt to keep the cost for unnecessary surgeries down, are encouraging and covering the costs for obtaining a second opinion. You are only outfitted with one reproductive system, so it is best to be certain that this surgery is needed. Exercise your right to obtain a second opinion without any guilt.

TALK WITH OTHER WOMEN
In addition to getting a second opinion, now is an excellent time to talk to other women who have had hysterectomies or those who are about to have one. The following resources may be useful in helping you contact women who have had or who are about to have a hysterectomy:

1. Your personal physican (since this is a surgery that he/she

performs, there should be no problem with getting a few names to contact)

2. Local women's health centers
3. Local chapter of Resolve, Inc. (if there is no chapter of Resolve in your area, contact the national headquarters listed in the appendix)
4. Contact the Endometriosis Association (names of women in your area who have had hysterectomies are available)
5. Contact local therapists who advertise focusing on women's issues (some therapists offer pre- and posthysterectomy workshops that may be useful to you)

If you are able to make contact with someone who has already had a hysterectomy, you can pool information and ask questions about her experience. If you make contact with someone about to have the surgery, then perhaps the two of you can pool energies and resources to accomplish the necessary research.

You now have all the information necessary to make an informed decision. Talk everything over with a close friend, partner or spouse, and then make a decision that you can live with. This surgery is not reversible, so it is important to be absolutely certain that this is what YOU think is best.

CHAPTER TWO

Laying the Groundwork

The first step in this process is to make certain that you have the best physician possible to handle your specific problem. Unfortunately, most of us take more care in selecting a brand of exercising shoes than we do in choosing our physicians. As informed consumers, it is important to get the best qualified, compassionate, ethical and compatible physician possible. There are several areas to investigate to assure that you are hiring the best person to handle your problem.

GUIDELINES TO DETERMINE
COMPETENCE AND COMPATIBILITY

1. Prior to your first appointment with the physician, determine what his/her credentials are. For help in doing this, refer to the Physician Evaluation Form, Section One—Credentials.
2. Check with friends and business associates who have had dealings with the physician you are considering. Find out what their experiences have been and what their opinion is of this doctor's medical ability.
3. Make certain to determine what his/her specialty is. Gynecologists are not all the same. Within each medical area there are numerous subspecialties. The following is a loose representation of subspecialties within the gynecology field:

   A general practice usually handles the day-to-day routine gynecological care of women. This covers the menstrual cycle and any problems connected with the cycle: family planning, pregnancies, vaginal infections, urology and some surgeries.

An oncology practice is usually limited to surgery of the pelvic area because of tumors (benign and malignant).

An endocrinology practice is usually limited to women with infertility problems and women who are experiencing difficulties after menopause, such as hot flashes, vaginal dryness and night sweats.

These categories may differ depending on your location. Metropolitan areas tend to have a larger number of physicians in subspecialties than rural areas. Nevertheless, it is important to determine your physician's strengths prior to making a decision about hiring him/her.

4. Immediately following your first visit, complete the remaining portion of the Physician Evaluation Form.
5. Evaluate all of the information gathered and make a decision whether or not this doctor is right for you.

Being an informed consumer is the appropriate role for a responsible adult to take. In order to make an intelligent decision you will need answers to many questions. Remember, your reluctance to investigate thoroughly might affect the quality of care you receive. A hysterectomy is very serious surgery. If the condition you have is severe enough to warrant such major surgery, it will be in your best interest to have the best possible person working on your body to ensure a positive outcome.

The Physician Evaluation Form is a tool designed to determine whether a particular physician is right for you. It consists of questions regarding credentials, communication, compassion and fees and services. Possible answers are provided, as well as a scoring system. While it is important to get answers to the questions in the form, there is no need to be combative or confrontational in doing so.

PHYSICIAN EVALUATION FORM

This evaluation form is divided into four sections:

1. Credentials
2. Communication
3. Compassion
4. Fees and Services

CREDENTIALS
(to be completed prior to the first visit)

1. What type of practice is the physician involved in?

	Points
hospital-based office	10
one specialty group	10
multispecialty group	8
informal association with others	8
alone	5

Answer = 10 points. A doctor who specializes and is part of a one specialty or hospital group is going to be aware of the most recent developments in his/her field of expertise. He/she will also be subject to ongoing review and scrutiny by fellow doctors within the group.

Answer = 8 points. A doctor who practices with a group which specializes in a variety of subspecialties of gynecology is not only a good generalist, but also a good resource person. He/she will probably know a person within the group who's more than competent to handle your problem.

Answer = 5 points. While informal association with others or practicing alone is not indicative of an underqualified physician, it might be in your best interest to enlist the services of a health care provider who is more immersed in the gynecological community.

2. What is this physician's status with regard to Board Certification? Board Certification means that a physician has met requirements with regard to training and in addition has passed written and oral examina-

tions administered by his/her colleagues. This person is judged to be intellectually competent.

	Points
board certified in specialty	10
board eligible	5
no longer board certified	1

Answer = 10 points. The term Board Certified means a physician has met course and residency requirements and passed oral and written examinations administered by other doctors. This physician is considered skilled in a particular area of medicine. You can check a physician's credentials through your local library in some areas. Ask for the Directory of Medical Specialists. This directory lists only those doctors who are Board Certified. The American Medical Directory is also a source to check a physician's credentials; however, it lists all members who belong to the American Medical Association whether they are Board Certified or not. If your local library does not have either of these reference guides then contact the American College of Obstetricians and Gynecologists, 600 Maryland Avenue, S.W., Washington, D.C. 20037. This group will provide you with referrals to Board Certified gynecologists in your area.

Answer = 5 points. The term Board Eligible refers to a physician who has completed course and residency requirements in a specialty, but has not taken the oral and written examinations. The Board Eligible physician may be as capable and qualified as the Board Certified physician, but it is more to his/her credit to be Certified than not. If you are otherwise comfortable with this doctor and think him/her capable, don't worry about the certification or lack thereof.

Answer = 1 point. If the doctor is no longer Board Certified, you need to find out why. Get a specific answer to this question, and then decide to continue with this doctor or not.

3. What type of hospital is this physician affiliated with?

	Points
university or medical school hospital	10
member of teaching staff of medical school	10
on staff at hospital with 200 or more beds	8

on staff at hospital with fewer than 200 beds	4
no hospital affiliation	1

Answer = 10 points.

Answer = 8 points. A physician who is on staff at a teaching hospital is probably one who has shown exemplary skill and knowledge and is respected by his/her colleagues.

Answer = 4 points. A physician who is on staff at a small hospital may certainly be as competent and capable as the physician practicing at the larger facility, but more care should be exercised in checking credentials.

Answer = 1 point. Ask the physician why he/she has no hospital affiliation. Perhaps he/she intends to refer you to someone else.

OVERALL SCORING

25-30 points—This physician has excellent credentials! He/she has the skills and knowledge to handle your case appropriately.

20-24 points—This physician, although not perfect, is certainly equipped in terms of knowledge and skill to give you good care.

below 20 points—This physician falls below average in the credential category. It would be in your best interest to consider another physician.

COMMUNICATION

1. Does the physician take a complete history and keep complete records?

	Points
full history	10
partial history	6
no history	0

Answer = 10 points. A full history involves getting information from you regarding various childhood diseases, problems, diseases and disorders that have occurred during your life, pregnancy history (including miscarriages, abortions and stillbirths), as well as a family history of illnesses (cancer, diabetes, heart disease, high blood pressure, phlebitis, anemia, etc.). Information regarding your lifestyle (use of tobacco, alcohol, recreational drugs), prescription drugs you are taking, allergies and finally a full description of the problem that brings you to your physician now. It is necessary to get a full history so that the physician has a better understanding of your physiological history and predispositions.

Answer = 6 points. If the presenting symptoms are severe, sometimes the doctor will postpone or omit taking a full history and address the acute problems. Be sure to present your doctor with a complete history at a subsequent visit. It is as much your responsibility as it is his/hers to get this information into your medical record.

Answer = 0 points. You are in serious trouble if no questions are asked! Your input and information regarding health problems are necessary for the physician making a diagnosis. Perhaps you should find another physician.

2. Does he/she really listen and hear what you are saying?

	Points
yes	10
not certain	2
no	0

Answer = 10 points. A doctor who listens to his/her patient carefully often finds out not only the physiological symptoms, but the psychological response to specific health problems. Such a doctor is in a better position to make a diagnosis and suggest a course of treatment than one who doesn't listen.

Answer = 2 points. A doctor who doesn't listen can be difficult if not impossible to work with. If you settle for a physician like this you run the risk of receiving inadequate care. You would be better off seeking out another physician.

3. How are diagnostic procedures explained?

	Points
diagnostic procedures are explained completely, risks or side effects that may be involved are discussed and diagrams are drawn when appropriate	10

diagnostic procedures are quickly explained in
   language not easily understood by the layperson
   and no mention of risks or side effects is made   7
diagnostic procedures are ordered and you are
   instructed to have them performed   2

Answer = 10 points. A doctor who takes time to explain your problem, suggested course of treatment and any risks involved is worthy of your trust. Your physician's commitment to full disclosure will put you in the best position to make an informed decision.

Answer = 7 points. Physicians are often under the impression that patients do not want to hear about risks. If your physician falls into this category, be assertive! Ask for more specifics regarding your condition and proposed method of treatment and ask what the risks are.

Answer = 2 points. Stop! Before having any diagnostic work performed request more information. Remember, this is your body "on the line"—handle it with care.

4. How are questions and fears handled?

                                                         Points
physician makes an effort to answer questions
   completely and address fears expressed   10
physician annoyed at questions, but answers
   grudgingly   6
physician refuses to answer questions   0

Answer = 10 points. Most physicians expect patients to have questions, and usually set aside time after the physical examination to answer questions, concerns and apprehensions.

Answer = 6 points. If your physician seems annoyed, call him/her on it. Explain that you understand about busy schedules and time limitations, but that it is equally important to you to have your questions answered satisfactorily.

Answer = 0 points. Find another doctor immediately! There is no excuse for this sort of treatment.

5. Do you understand what your physician is saying?

	Points
yes, although medical terminology is used, the explanation is always in plain English	10
vaguely, the physician uses many words that you don't understand and few words that you do understand	8
no, it is all a mystery to you	2

Answer = 10 points. This is what every responsible patient hopes for: a physician who speaks in understandable terms.

Answer = 8 points. If your physician is in this category, meet him/her halfway. Go to a medical library (located at a medical school or hospital) and research your disease. Familiarize yourself with the jargon and find out what it all means. This will take some time, but it is certainly better than being in the dark. If you continue to have difficulty understanding, simply ask him/her to explain.

Answer = 2 points. Speak up! Tell your doctor that you don't understand. Hopefully, you'll both make an effort to understand each other. However, if mutual understanding never comes, it would be in your best medical interest to find another doctor.

6. How is the office run?

	Points
friendly, warm, efficient office personnel; appointments are kept on time (the rule as opposed to the exception)	10
cold, clinical, impersonal staff and office; waiting is the standard operating procedure	7
staff seems friendly and caring, but physician is always behind and not as concerned about you as is his/her staff	5
messy, cluttered office, staffed with unkempt, uncaring personnel	0

Answer = 10 points. The operation of this office inspires confidence that you'll be in good hands.

Answer = 7 points. It appears that your time is not respected or viewed as being as valuable as the physician's. When waiting becomes the rule as opposed to the exception, it is time to speak up.

Answer = 5 points. While it is comforting to have a warm and friendly staff supporting the patient, if the physician doesn't show as much concern for you, then there's a problem. The physician, not his/her support staff, is responsible for your care. Be leery of this sort of situation.

Answer = 0 points. This has all the warning signs of a substandard office with a physician who probably provides substandard care. Exit immediately!

OVERALL SCORING

45-60 points—Your physician has excellent communication skills. A partnership relationship is definitely possible with this doctor.

36-44 points—Your physician may need help from you in determining how to meet your needs, but this doctor does have the capacity to be a partner in your health care.

below 36 points—This physician is going to represent a challenge. Take a closer look at your need or desire to have this person as your health care provider.

COMPASSION

1. How does the physician interact with you?

	Points
warm, concerned and interested, listens and attempts to interact with you by explaining and answering questions and concerns	10
intellectually competent, but displays minimal warmth	8
distant, makes no effort to slow down long enough to recognize that the disease he/she is trying to treat and cure has a person attached to it	2

Answer = 10 points. Most of us want our doctor to interact with us in this manner. This is the optimal situation.

Answer = 8 points. Perhaps this doctor could use a strong dose of warmth, but if he/she is otherwise competent maybe you can achieve a good working relationship.

Answer = 2 points. Lacking warmth is one thing, but the absence of compassion and the presence of distance is a definite warning. This doctor may not be suitable for you.

FEES AND SERVICES

1. Is the physician willing to discuss fees?

	Points
yes	10
no	0

Answer = 10 points. Fees are important. It is necessary to work out any problems and difficulties before any major costs are incurred.

Answer = 0 points. There is no excuse for not discussing this subject.

2. Is the physician accessible after regular office hours?

	Points
yes, willing to make telephone contact or house call in case of emergency	10
no, unwilling to communicate after regular office hours; answering service operator refers you to the emergency room of the nearest hospital	2

Answer = 10 points. When you are in the midst of a crisis, it is necessary to be able to contact your physician for emergency services or to answer questions. Responsible physicians are normally available to their patients. You must be careful, however not to abuse this service with nonemergency calls.

Answer = 2 points. Find out why your physician is inaccessible. Determine if you can live with this aspect of his/her delivery of services to you and make a decision accordingly.

OVERALL SCORING
(for Compassion and Fees and Services Categories)

26-30 points—If your physician is in this category he/she has above average compassion for patients.

20-25 points—Your physician has an average amount of compassion, probably enough to have a comfortable, effective working relationship with you.

below 20 points—Compassion is not one of this physician's strengths. If this characteristic is not important to you, this doctor will probably be adequate for your needs.

HOW TO CREATE A PHYSICIAN–PATIENT PARTNERSHIP

Assessing a physician's credentials, competence and compatibility to work with you is only the first step in developing a physician–patient partnership. Your next step is to continue to actively participate in obtaining help for yourself. This may be accomplished in three ways:

1. Establish with the physician what your role in this partnership is going to be.
2. Be specific about reporting your symptoms.
3. Be intelligent enough to ask questions and discuss any fears and apprehensions.

Establishing a partnership relationship with your physician is not the easiest thing in the world to do because it is a relatively new manner of approaching health care delivery. For years we as patients have been advised to put our bodies in the hands of "Doctor God," who will perform miracles on our ill bodies. Doctors and patients alike bring this kind of thinking to the relationship making a partnership relationship possible, but initially difficult to achieve. When you enter into this relationship you will come with your own set of expectations. In general, it is reasonable to expect:

• The doctor should be knowledgeable about health and illness and able to recognize the difference between the two.
• The doctor should be helpful. To be helpful means to understand the nature of the symptoms and to have a clear course of action for investigating and finding a solution for the problem.

- The doctor will allow you to participate in the process involving diagnosis and treatment to as great a degree as possible.
- The doctor will adhere to a "full disclosure" relationship. (Some physicians are hesitant to initiate a full disclosure relationship because patients are sometimes frightened by the facts of their case. Sometimes doctors will make the decision to withhold information because of their uncertainty as to how the patient will handle the information. It is your responsibility to make your need for full disclosure known up front.)

KEEPING A HEALTH JOURNAL

Since physicians are not magicians, it is important to provide accurate, specific information about yourself whenever possible. The most efficient way to handle this is by means of a health journal (see table 1). Such a journal doesn't need to be fancy, only complete and efficient. A simple notebook will be adequate. Be certain to include important symptoms such as: temperature, weight gain/loss, bleeding (severity and color), pain (sharp or dull, constant or intermittent), nausea, vomiting, etc. Be sure to keep track of any medications that you are

TABLE 1

	Pain	Bleeding	Nausea/ Vomiting	Temp.	Other
Sunday	sharp intermittent	light brownish	none	100.2	painful sex, depression
Monday	sharp intermittent	light brownish	none	98.6	none
Tuesday	sharp intermittent	medium brown/red	nausea	100.2	dizzy
Wednesday	sharp continuous	medium/heavy dark red	nausea	101.4	dizzy/tired
Thursday	sharp continuous	heavy bright red	vomiting	101.6	fainted twice
Friday	unbearable	heavy bright red	vomiting	102.4	dizzy
Saturday	unbearable	heavy bright red	vomiting	103.0	dizzy

taking (prescription or other) during this period. It will also be helpful to include any emotional stress occurring in your life. The sample page of the health journal as presented in table 1 represents a woman with progressively worsening symptoms. She notified her physician on Wednesday and was hospitalized on Thursday. The journal provides both doctor and patient with specific information that is sometimes lost to memory.

CHAPTER   THREE

The Hospital Experience

Once you have decided that surgery is necessary, the next step is to prepare for the hospital experience. Many of us don't do so because we don't know how, or what to expect, and the result is often surprise and sometimes fear of the hospital procedures. Hysterectomy is major surgery psychologically as well as physiologically. To ensure the most positive results, it helps to take some responsibility for your hospital experience. There are five aspects that women should address regarding hospitalization for a hysterectomy:

1. admission procedures
2. psychological preparation
3. spiritual considerations
4. legal precautions
5. preoperative preparations

ADMISSION PROCEDURES AND TESTS

Admission refers to the administrative and physiologic procedures required by most hospitals prior to any medical treatment. The most important piece of information to bring is your insurance card or number. This is necessary because the admissions secretary will have to verify that you are covered by insurance. If, for some reason, you are not covered by insurance, the hospital will require an advance deposit or full payment of the estimated charges for your hospital stay. The physician's fee for performing a hysterectomy averages between

$1,700 and $2,300. This fee may be a bit higher if more extensive surgery is performed. As for hospital costs, it really depends on where you are located geographically, but you can expect to pay between $4,000 and $7,000.

The name and address of the person to contact in case of emergency will also be required at this time. You will sign an admission form (figure 3.1), as well as other forms regarding the release of responsibility for stolen personal items (figure 3.2). An identification bracelet will be placed on your wrist containing your hospital number as well as your name and birth date. You will then be assigned a room and a hospital volunteer will escort you to it.

Once you are in your room, a nurse will come and take a brief history. She will then take your temperature, blood pressure and pulse, and explain what is going to happen to you during the next few days. Some of the tests and procedures commonly performed are:

chest X-ray—required of all patients admitted unless you've had one within the last six months

standard lab work—urinalysis and cbc (complete blood count) are necessary to help determine whether or not there is an infection present as well as any other abnormalities

blood type, cross and match—determines your blood type in the event that you need a transfusion

IVP (intravenous pyelogram)—This test is usually performed on patients who are undergoing extensive abdominal surgery. A small quantity of iodine is injected intravenously to provide contrast to the kidneys, ureters and bladder. This procedure is painless. However, if you have an allergy to iodine inform the doctor before the test is performed. This test allows the physician to spot irregularities in the functioning of the kidneys, ureters and bladder.

barium enema—This test is performed whenever there is extensive surgery in the abdominal cavity, especially if the intestines are involved in the problem. Barium (a white, chalky substance) is introduced rectally into the lower intestinal tract and its movement through the intestinal tract is carefully studied. Although this procedure is not painful, it is somewhat uncomfortable. If you can focus your attention on relaxing your muscles, the test will be tolerable.

vital signs—This is a procedure in which your temperature, blood pressure and pulse are taken every four hours. These indicate how your body is functioning. While it may seem unnecessary to take vitals prior to surgery, this information will provide the caregiving staff with a baseline of what is normal for you.

doctor's orders—Without these orders, very little will happen. It is standard operating procedure for the attending physician to provide medical staff with written orders regarding your care. This practice can be carried to the extreme, but the requirement is a sound one and exists for everyone's protection.

visitors—The rules regarding visitors vary from hospital to hospital. Some facilities allow unlimited visits from a spouse, parent or close friend. Other facilities adhere strictly to the posted hours. If you have a problem with the preset visiting arrangements, discuss it with your physician or the charge nurse. There is a good chance that most problems can be worked out. If you are not successful with this approach, contact the hospital's Patient Advocate office. A Patient Advocate is a person usually employed by the hospital. He/she acts as a liaison between the hospital and the patient, addresses any problems, questions or difficulties that you may be experiencing and tries to resolve them. You do not have to choose the advocate employed by the hospital. A spouse, parent or a good friend may also act in your interests.

After the preliminary testing is completed, a physician will take a complete history and do a physical examination. Be sure to disclose everything while he/she is taking your history. Some women feel embarrassed to talk about the number of pregnancies, miscarriages and abortions they experienced, others are ashamed or embarrassed to talk about their recreational use of drugs. Information that you may be reticent to provide may be vital to ensuring the best medical care. The physician is not there to judge you, but to help heal you. If you happen to be in a teaching facility, residents will probably ask for your history several times. If you find this overwhelming and/or unnecessary, say so and ask the person requesting the information to explain why it is really necessary to repeat your story.

PSYCHOLOGICAL PREPARATION

Because facing a hysterectomy can be an emotionally wrenching experience, you would be wise to consider the process of psychologically preparing for the hospital stay. Here are three things that might help you:

> *friends*—Compassionate, loving friends are vital to your emotional well-being. You may find, however, that some people whom you are particularly close to and on whom you normally depend for company and sympathy are just the wrong people to have around at this time—perhaps because they are so upset by your illness, or by illness in general, that they make you feel worse rather than better. On the other hand, you may find that other people, ones you have not considered terribly close previously, have surprising reserves of patience, calmness and intelligent concern. It is hard to pick your company cold-bloodedly at any time, let alone when you are facing surgery, and you certainly will not want to hurt your friends' feelings, but you will be better off if you can avoid depending for comfort on those who can't give it, and still better off if you find someone who can give you comfort and can perhaps even advocate for you if necessary.

> *accoutrements*—Most hospital rooms are not decorated in accordance with your personal tastes. Therefore, a few items from home will help you feel more comfortable. Here are some suggestions:
> • pictures, posters or wall hangings
> • small, inexpensive radio with earplug
> • a pillow
> • toiletries and a sanitary belt
> • night gown, robe and slippers

- stuffed animal (don't be ashamed)
- books or magazines
- anything else that would make you more comfortable

reassurance—If you have any fears whatsoever, address them before surgery. Patient teaching and reassuring are part of the nursing staff's job. Nurses are more than willing to answer your questions, as time permits, of course. If a question is best answered by your physician, the nurse will inform him/her on your behalf.

SPIRITUAL CONSIDERATIONS

Spiritual needs are often overlooked and neglected. At this time you will want to utilize all resources for support and comfort. Ministers, rabbis and priests, as well as the solitude of prayer or meditation can be helpful during this time.

Perhaps you can arrange for your minister or other members of your religious community to help meet your spiritual needs. Even if you haven't had time to arrange such visits in advance you can feel free to take the opportunity to discuss your feelings with the hospital chaplain. Within the first day or two the chaplain will stop by your room to introduce him/herself. You'll be asked what religious preference you have, if any, if you want anyone contacted (a particular minister, family member or friend) and if it is all right for the hospital chaplain to drop by to visit you again. Even if you are not particularly religious it might be nice to have a visit from a compassionate person who knows the hospital ropes and can intervene for you if necessary.

LEGAL PRECAUTIONS

Patient's Bill of Rights—As a medical consumer, you have an obligation to familiarize yourself with the Patient's Bill of Rights (figure 3.3). All hospitals should have a copy in the admissions and patient advocate's office. It is not sufficient to merely be aware of your rights as a patient— you or your advocate should be willing to exercise those rights should it become necessary.

Informed Consent—To be capable of making an intelligent decision it is first necessary to have all pertinent facts. In this situation the pertinent facts are:

- an explanation of your condition;
- an explanation of the procedure to be performed;
- an explanation of alternatives to the suggested procedure if there are any;
- a description of the benefits to be expected (this does not imply a warranty);
- a description of the risks and side effects of the procedure;
- an opportunity to ask questions;
- an understanding that you are not being coerced into compliance and that you may reject treatment if you change your mind.

You will be asked to sign an "Informed Consent" form (figure 3.4: form 1, 2, or 4). Your signature on this form authorizes the anesthesiologist and surgical team to provide service. You don't have to agree to all the conditions as listed on the form. For example, if you would prefer not to have your surgery photographed, simply cross out the line or lines that pertain to photographing the surgery (form 1). Or if you are adamant about your physician performing the surgery as opposed to the senior resident, be sure to write in your physician's name (form 4). The best way to protect your interests is to spell everything out legally. While it is your physician's responsibility to provide you with expert care, it is your responsibility to set limits and/or restrictions if necessary. Signing a consent form does not lock you into a decision. You always have the option to rescind the consent.

PREOPERATIVE PREPARATION

Once the routine testing is completed and the consent forms are signed, the presurgical preparation will begin. The following is a general list of procedures which may be part of your preparation for the hysterectomy:

Approximately twenty-four hours prior to surgery

- you'll be placed on a clear liquid diet (this diet helps decrease the amount of waste material in your intestinal tract; this is important because your intestinal functioning will be limited immediately following surgery);
- you'll be given citrate of magnesia and an enema;
- the areas to be exposed during surgery will be shaved;
- you'll be asked to douche;
- the anesthesiologist will speak to you about his/her role in your surgery, you'll be asked about your respiratory history (asthma, allergies, etc.). If you have fears about being "put under," speak to him/her about those fears at this time;
- your physician will order a sedative in case you have trouble getting to sleep.

The day of surgery

- an intravenous line (IV) will be started (a small catheter is inserted into the vein in the wrist or the forearm) to provide pre- and postoperative medication and/or anesthesia;
- you'll be asked to remove dentures, glasses, etc.;
- your identification bracelet will be checked;
- you will be given a sedative injection;
- you will be transferred to the pre-op waiting/holding suite;
- you will be transferred to the operating room.

UNDERSTANDING THE SURGICAL PROCEDURE

The word hysterectomy comes from the Greek word *hystero,* which, according to Urdang's Dictionary of Medical Terms, refers to the womb and secondly to hysteria, and *ectomy,* the removal of. It is interesting that hysteria is a part of the meaning of hysterectomy because Freud suggested that hysteria was a result of frustrated libidinous impulses in women. This theory would support why early physicians doubted the validity of women's complaints in regard to their female organs. However, as we have developed and progressed scientifically and culturally, medical attitudes have changed. And today, while there is still some reticence toward accepting pelvic complaints as valid, most qualified physicians understand many of the intricacies of the functioning of the female reproductive system. Hysterectomy refers to the surgical removal of the uterus. This removal can be achieved vaginally or abdominally depending on why the surgery is being performed.

Abdominal hysterectomy procedures account for approximately 70 percent of all hysterectomies, and total hysterectomies account for approximately 95 percent of all procedures.[8] A *total hysterectomy* involves the removal of the cervix and the uterus. A *subtotal procedure* is one in which the cervix remains intact. In a *radical hysterectomy,* the lymph nodes, supporting ligaments and upper portion of the vagina are cut and removed. The ligaments are attached to the vaginal cuff, so the normal depth of the vagina is maintained.

Sometimes, one or both of the fallopian tubes and ovaries are removed. This procedure is called *unilateral or bilateral salpingo-oophorectomy.* As long as one ovary remains, menopause should not occur. However, if both ovaries are removed, "surgical menopause" will occur (see Chapter 5).

Abdominal hysterectomy usually takes several hours to complete depending on the nature of the disease, the severity of the disease and the organs to be removed. The more severe cases of a particular disease often require a more extensive, intricate approach and a longer operating time. There will be a vertical scar following an abdominal hysterectomy. If you had surgery prior to the hysterectomy, the surgeon will probably cut where you have been cut before, thereby leaving one scar. The incision will probably be closed by use of staples (this sounds barbaric, but is the most efficient and safe method of closing this type of incision). Total hospitalization time for an abdominal hysterectomy without complications is approximately seven to ten days.

Vaginal hysterectomy involves the removal of the uterus and the cervix only, through the vagina. Physicians make use of this method when there is no medical problem in the abdominal cavity and therefore no reason to expose those organs to the trauma of surgery. Vaginal hysterectomy has several contraindications such as: the presence of pelvic inflammatory disease, ovarian tumors, an enlarged uterus (large means the size of a twelve to fourteen week fetus), endometriosis, previous pelvic radiation therapy, invasive cervical cancer, and a narrow vagina (this would make this type of surgery nearly impossible). Abdominal hysterectomy has no contraindications other than the usual contraindications to any surgical procedure. Vaginal hysterectomy takes approximately one or two hours to complete, barring complications.

There will be a small scar following vaginal hysterectomy, located where your cervix was located. However, it will be internal, and visible only to your gynecologist.

RISKS AND COMPLICATIONS

Although the purpose of any surgical procedure is to correct problems that affect the quality of life, surgery itself comes with its own set of possible problems and complications. The most common complications reported for vaginal and abdominal hysterectomy are:

Infection—Infection is more frequent after vaginal hysterectomy than abdominal hysterectomy. These infections are usually treated with antibiotics.

Urinary tract—Urinary tract infections, urinary retention, and stress incontinence occur more frequently with vaginal hysterectomies. Urinary tract infections are treated with antibiotics. Stress incontinence can be improved through muscle-toning exercises (Kegel exercises, discussed in Chapter 7).

Hemorrhage—Hemorrhaging may occur immediately after surgery or a week or two after surgery. It occurs most often in younger women after a vaginal hysterectomy.

Bowel obstruction—This complication occurs usually after abdominal hysterectomy. The more common symptoms are constipation, vomiting, abdominal distension and lack of bowel sounds. It takes approximately three to five days for normal bowel function to return following abdominal hysterectomy. If there appears to be an abnormal obstruction in the bowel, a nasogastric tube (a small tube inserted through the nostril and into the stomach) will be used to withdraw the blockage.

Thrombophlebitis—This is a condition involving inflammation and clotting of the deep veins of the lower extremities which usually occurs following abdominal hysterectomy. This problem is more common in obese women. The usual care for this condition is leg elevation, and use of anti-embolism stockings.

Pulmonary—Pulmonary complications occur more frequently after abdominal hysterectomy. Pneumonia and pulmonary embolism are the most common problems. They are prevented by the use of respiration therapy, Heparin (an anticoagulant drug) injections, and walking soon after surgery (within twenty-four hours).

Bladder damage—Bladder damage occurs most frequently in vaginal hysterectomies. Sometimes the bladder is nicked or cut in the process of removing the uterus. If the damage to the bladder is noted at the time of surgery, the surgeon can repair it. Otherwise a fistula (a hole or opening) may form. If this happens, surgery will be required to repair the damage.

Wound separation—Wound separation occurs more often with abdominal hysterectomies. Resuturing or stapling of the wound is required.

Risk of anesthesia—With any general surgery there is always a risk of allergic reaction to anesthesia. All allergies should be reported and discussed with the anesthesiologist prior to surgery.

UNDERSTANDING THE STAGES OF RECOVERY

The recovery period begins in the operating room, immediately following surgery, and continues until your convalescence is complete. There are four important stages to your recovery process:

Transfer—involves transferring you from the operating room to the recovery room without causing injury.

Monitoring 1—involves close monitoring of vital signs and stabilization of the patient by the recovery room staff. Vital signs are usually taken every fifteen minutes postoperatively for the first hour, every

thirty minutes until stable, thereafter every four hours.

Monitoring 2—involves the continued monitoring of the woman's condition by the floor nursing staff until time of discharge. Hysterectomy patients are encouraged to:

- Turn, cough and deep breathe at regular intervals (every two to three hours during the first twenty-four hours postoperatively, less frequently thereafter). If an abdominal hysterectomy was performed, it may be necessary to support the abdomen with a pillow when coughing. The coughing, turning and deep breathing regimen is necessary because anesthesia increases the secretions in your lungs and these secretions must be coughed out to prevent pneumonia.
- Walking is also an important part of the recovery process. The nurse will teach you how to get out of bed with a minimum of discomfort. Once out of bed, you should attempt a short walk, perhaps with some assistance at first. Walking improves circulation, muscle tone, lung expansion and bowel functions. Although it may be uncomfortable at first, stick with it. The results will aid in your overall recovery.
- Wear those support stockings given to you after your surgery. These stockings as well as injections of Heparin will help prevent thrombophlebitis (blood clots in the veins).
- Alert the nurse to any excess bleeding. It is normal to have a moderate amount of vaginal bleeding, but if you suspect a problem, let the nursing staff or physician know about it.
- Accurately report your pain. The amount of pain medication administered will depend on the type of surgery and your tolerance for pain. This is a very tricky issue, because some patients attempt to hide their pain or ignore it. It is normal to experience pain following surgery and this pain should decrease in severity after a few days. If your level of pain doesn't change, speak to your physician. The doctor depends on you to assess the effectiveness of pain medication. If a particular drug is not making you more comfortable, speak up. Another drug may be more effective in alleviating your pain.

- Keep in mind that the primary purpose of pain medication is to decrease the amount of pain you are experiencing. It is not meant to transport you to an eternal altered state of consciousness. If the medication does not make you more comfortable you should of course speak up. You should also report to the nursing staff if a drug is too strong for your pain levels. As your pain levels decrease, the amount and type of medication will change as well.
- Follow the prescribed diet. Your diet will progress from clear liquids to a soft diet to a regular diet. The rate of progression usually depends on your rate of recovery and the return of full bowel functioning.
- Schedule your visitors. Considering the strenuous (physical and psychological) process that you've undergone, it may be wise to consider whether or not to limit the number of visitors and the timing of their visits. It is certainly important to have contact with those people who are special to you so that they may see for themselves that you are okay. It is also important for you to do your part to ensure a total recovery. Some tips on handling visitors:

  Be up front with them. Explain that a short visit (twenty minutes or less) is definitely welcome, but that you aren't yet up for anything longer.

  Encourage friends to call before coming. This allows you the option of postponing a visit if you're too tired and it gives you time to wash your face, brush your teeth, comb your hair, etc., thus affording you maximum dignity.

  If there is a specific time that you are particularly lonely (meal time or mid-afternoon, for example), try to schedule visits for these times.

  If your husband, boyfriend or special friend visits at a particular time, remember to keep that time clear. Spread your visitors throughout the day if possible. You'll be less tired and less lonely if you do.

  Your job is to recover, not to entertain. Many of us enjoy making our guests comfortable, but this is quite a different situation. Your

visitors should be there to help entertain, comfort and love you, not the reverse.

If visitors become tedious, asking extremely personal or sensitive questions, begin telling you how awful you look or anything else equally offensive, thank them for coming to visit and explain that you are still recovering and need your rest. Sometimes friends are uncomfortable seeing someone they care about in less than optimal condition and this discomfort can result in inappropriate comments.

- Accept the blues as part of the healing process. For some women, the third or fourth day following surgery is extremely difficult. Some women describe themselves feeling sad, weepy, angry and/or frustrated. The cards, flowers and visits begin to drop off, hospital policy dictates your routine (meals, medication, visitors, etc.) and you may become tired of it all. You may feel trapped in an antiseptic fishbowl, because although you're beginning to feel better, you are not yet ready to make a break for freedom. Allow yourself a good cry and a little self-pity. The quality of your life should improve steadily from this point on.
- Prepare yourself for going home. The trip home begins the final phase of your recovery. Up to this point, you have been carefully monitored and guided by the hospital health care team. You are now at a point in your recovery where you need less intensive care. Begin slowly to add activities to your daily routine until you have returned to a normal schedule. You may not have as much energy as you'd like, but remember that the healing process does take time.

Monitoring 3—Arrange for someone (spouse, relative or friend) to help you for a few days. Perhaps this person could help by preparing meals, doing the laundry, running the vacuum cleaner or just sitting with you and talking. If you can't arrange for such a person to assist you, forget about the household chores and have handy a list of restaurants that deliver. If you happen to be fortunate enough to have family who live locally, perhaps you could spend a week or so with them.

Figure 3.1

FINANCIAL AGREEMENT

I understand and accept that it is my duty to pay for any hospital charges for which I am billed by the University. I also understand that I will receive separate bill(s) for the professional care given to me by physician(s). I know that if I am given professional care by a physician who is an employee of the University, I will receive a bill from the University's Medical Faculty Associates. I also agree to pay those medical bills.

I give permission to my insurance provider(s), including Medicare and Medicaid, to directly pay   University for my care instead of paying me. I know that I will have to pay what my insurance does not pay or cover.

I agree to the University sending copies of my medical records (or information from my medical records) to my insurance provider(s) or other sources of payment, which may include my employer. I understand that this information will be sent when it is needed for payment of my medical bills. I release and forever discharge University, its employees and agents from any liability resulting from the release of my medical records or information from them for payment purposes.

I know that if I am a member of a Health Maintenance Organization (HMO), the HMO will only pay medical bills for care and treatment it agreed to pay for before the care or treatment is actually given or received. I understand that among those bills that I may have to pay are those for care and treatment I received without the advanced approval from the HMO.

I understand that any information I am given by the University as to the charges for the medical care and/or hospital stay or what my insurance company should pay of those charges is only an estimate. I understand and agree, therefore, that I am responsible for all medical bills even if they are higher than the estimate.

I know that if these medical bills are not paid on time, they may be turned over to an attorney for collection. If that happens, I understand and agree that I will have to pay the University's attorney's fee. This fee will be 15% of the amount that I owe.

I have read this contract and have had all of my questions about it answered. I understand the contract and I agree to its terms.

Patient _____(seal) Date_____
                (signature)

Responsible Party _____(seal) Date_____
(If other than Patient) (signature)

Witness _____(seal) Date_____

Figure 3.2

AUTHORIZATION FOR MEDICAL CARE AND TREATMENT
AUTHORIZATION FOR RELEASE OF MEDICAL RECORDS
TO THIRD-PARTY PAYERS
RELEASE OF RESPONSIBILITY FOR PERSONAL PROPERTY/VALUABLES

1. I have come to _____ Hospital for medical treatment. I ask the health care professionals at the Hospital to provide care and treatment for me as they feel is necessary. I consent to undergo routine tests and treatment as part of this care. I understand that I am free to ask a member of my health care team questions about any care, treatment or medicine I am to receive.

2. Because _____ Hospital is a teaching hospital, I understand that my health care team will be made up of hospital personnel and medical students in addition to my attending physician and his/her assistants and designees. Hospital personnel include, but are not limited to, nurses, technicians, interns, residents, and fellows.

3. I understand that as part of my care and treatment, samples of my blood, urine, stool and tissues may be removed from me from time to time. I permit the University to use any leftover blood, urine, stool and tissues for research. (If I do not want the University to so use leftover portions, I may stop the University from doing so by writing "no" in the following block and writing my initials after it _____ .) If additional samples are needed for the research, I will be asked at that time.

4. I am aware that the practice of medicine is not an exact science and admit that no one has given me any promises or guarantees about the result of any care or treatment I am to receive or examinations I am to undergo.

5. I agree to the University sending copies of my medical records (or information from my medical records) to my insurance provider(s) or other sources of payment, which may include my employer. I understand that this information will be sent when it is needed for payment of my medical bills. I release and forever discharge The _____ , its employees and agents from any liability resulting from the release of my medical records or information from them for payment purposes.

6. Release of Responsibility for Personal Property/Valuables: I understand that _____ University is not responsible for any personal property or valuables that I keep with me while I am in the Hospital. Personal property includes, but is not limited to, clothing, shoes and baggage. Valuables include, but are not limited to, money, credit cards, dentures, eyeglasses, hearing aids, and jewelry.

I understand that my property/valuables should be sent home with my family/friends and that I am responsible for the safekeeping of any items of property or valuables that I do keep with me. I also realize that valuables I cannot send home with family/friends may be stored with the Cashier's Office.

I desire to store my valuables.   ☐ YES   ☐ NO

AFFIRMATION

I have read this form and understand it. All of my questions about what it says have been answered. I am signing it of my own free will. I understand that by signing it, I am agreeing to it.

_____   _____
Signature of patient (or parent, legal guardian   *Date/Time*
or next-of-kin. Please indicate which.)

_____   _____
Witness to affirmation and signature   *Date/Time*

Figure 3.3

A PATIENT'S BILL OF RIGHTS

1. The patient has the right to considerate and respectful care.

2. The patient has the right to obtain from his physician complete current information concerning his diagnosis, treatment, and prognosis in terms the patient can be reasonably expected to understand.

3. The patient has the right to receive from his physician information necessary to give informed consent prior to the start of any procedure and/or treatment. Except in emergencies, such information for informed consent should include but not necessarily be limited to the specific procedure and/or treatment, the medically significant risks involved, and the probable duration of incapacitation.

4. The patient has the right to refuse treatment to the extent permitted by law, and to be informed of the medical consequences of his action.

5. The patient has the right to every consideration of his privacy concerning his own medical care program. Case discussion, consultation, examination, and treatment are confidential and should be conducted discreetly. Those not directly involved in his care must have the permission of the patient to be present.

6. The patient has the right to expect that all communications and records pertaining to his care should be treated as confidential.

7. The patient has the right to expect that within its capacity a hospital must make reasonable response to the request of a patient for service. . . . When medically permissible a patient may be transferred to another facility only after he has received complete information and explanation concerning the needs for and alternatives to such a transfer.

8. The patient has the right to obtain information as to any relationship of his hospital to other health care and educational institutions insofar as his care is concerned.

9. The patient has the right to be advised if the hospital proposes to engage in or perform human experimentation affecting his care or treatment. The patient has the right to refuse to participate in such research projects.

10. The patient has the right to expect reasonable continuity of care. He has the right to know in advance what appointment times and physicians are available and when. The patient has the right to expect that the hospital will provide a mechanism whereby he is informed by his physician or a delegate of the physician of the patient's continuing health.

Figure 3.4   Consent Forms

FORM 1
CONSENT TO OPERATION, ANESTHETICS,
AND OTHER MEDICAL SERVICES*

                                                                    A.M.
                        Date＿＿＿＿＿＿Time＿＿＿＿＿＿P.M.

1. I authorize the performance upon ＿＿＿＿＿＿＿＿＿＿＿＿＿＿＿
                                        (myself or name of patient)
of the following operation ＿＿＿＿＿＿＿＿＿＿＿＿＿＿＿＿＿＿
                                (state nature and extent of operation)
to be performed by or under the direction of Dr. ＿＿＿＿＿＿＿＿.

2. I consent to the performance of operations and procedures in addition to or different from those now contemplated, whether or not arising from presently unforeseen conditions, which the above-named doctor or his associates or assistants may consider necessary or advisable in the course of the operation.

3. I consent to the administration of such anesthetics as may be considered necessary or advisable by the physician responsible for this service, with the exception of ＿＿＿＿＿＿＿＿＿＿＿＿＿＿＿
                                (state "none," "spinal anesthesia," etc.)

4. The nature and purpose of the operation, possible alternative methods of treatment, the risks involved, the possible consequences, and the possibility of complications have been explained to me by Dr. ＿＿＿＿＿＿＿＿＿＿＿＿ and by ＿＿＿＿＿＿＿＿＿＿＿＿.

5. I acknowledge that no guarantee or assurance has been given by anyone as to the results that may be obtained.

6. I consent to the photographing or televising of the operations or procedures to be performed, including appropriate portions of my body, for medical, scientific or educational purposes, provided my identity is not revealed by the pictures or by descriptive texts accompanying them.

7. For the purpose of advancing medical education, I consent to the admittance of observers to the operating room.

8. I consent to the disposal by hospital authorities of any tissues or body parts which may be removed.

9. I am aware that sterility may result from this operation. I know that a sterile person is incapable of becoming a parent.

10. I acknowledge that all blank spaces on this document have been either completed or crossed off prior to my signing.

(CROSS OUT ANY PARAGRAPHS ABOVE WHICH DO NOT AP-PLY)

                        Signed ＿＿＿＿＿＿＿＿＿＿＿＿＿＿
                            (Patient or person authorized
                                to consent for patient)

Witness＿＿＿＿＿＿＿＿＿＿＿＿

*This is a general form of consent which will apply to various procedures by striking out the portions which are inapplicable.

FORM 2
CONSENT TO OPERATION, ANESTHETICS, AND
OTHER MEDICAL SERVICES (ALTERNATE FORM)*

A.M.
Date_____ Time_____ P.M.

1. I authorize the performance upon _____
(myself or name of patient)
of the following operation _____
(state name of operation)
to be performed under the direction of Dr. _____.
2. The following have been explained to me by Dr. _____:
A. The nature of the operation _____
(describe the operation)

_____

B. The purpose of the operation _____
(describe the purpose)

_____

C. The possible alternative methods of treatment _____

_____
(describe the alternative methods)
D. The possible consequences of the operation _____

_____
(describe the possible consequences)
E. The risks involved _____
(describe the risks involved)

_____

F. The possibility of complications _____

_____
(describe the possible complications)
3. I have been advised of the serious nature of the operation and have been advised that if I desire a further and more detailed explanation of any of the foregoing or further information about the possible risks or complications of the above listed operation it will be given to me.
4. I do not request a further and more detailed listing and explanation of any of the items listed in paragraph 2.

Signed _____
*(Patient or person authorized
to consent for patient)*

Witness_____

*This is an alternate form of consent which will provide an opportunity for the physician or hospital to include a detailed disclosure of the operation. The appropriate paragraphs from Form 1 may be added to this form.

FORM 4
CONSENT TO OPERATION, ANESTHETICS, AND OTHER MEDICAL SERVICES AT TEACHING INSTITUTION*

A.M.

Date_____ Time_____ P.M.

1. I authorize the performance upon _____
(myself or name of patient)

of the following operation _____
(state name of operation)

2. I understand that the operation is to be performed at _____
_____, a teaching institution.

3. I understand that the operation, the medical services rendered in conjunction with the operation, and the post-operative care are to be performed and rendered by those individuals selected and deemed qualified by the teaching medical staff of the

_____

(name of the institution)

Signed _____

*(Patient or person authorized
to consent for patient)*

Witness_____

*The appropriate paragraphs from Form 1 may be added to this form.

The Need to Mourn

UNDERSTANDING THE STAGES OF GRIEF

Now that you have settled in at home, you'll find yourself with more time to go over what has happened to you—the actual physical procedure and the emotional impact it has begun to have on your life. And, because you'll be alone most of the time while you are recuperating, it will be somewhat difficult to avoid these thoughts.

It is important to understand that it is normal to mourn the loss of your reproductive capability. It is equally important to recognize that each woman will grieve in her own way. Mourning always occurs at some level of consciousness. For some women it may take the form of a feeling of sadness about the need for hysterectomy, and for others it may take on some of the characteristic stages of grief, and some women may give the appearance of not grieving at all. Don't worry about whether or not you are grieving in the right way. There is no best way to grieve. Individual women should mourn this loss in a way that is appropriate and useful for them.

Grieving is a natural process. It is helpful to understand the various stages of grief. They are:

> denial
> anger
> bargaining
> depression
> acceptance

Grieving actually begins, at least to some extent, prior to the hysterectomy. In fact, it often begins at the time of diagnosis or at the time when a woman decides that hysterectomy is the best option. The stages of grief are not absolutes. They are simply meant to serve as signposts for emotions you might experience during this time. You may experience one or more of these stages, but it is not mandatory for you to experience them all.

DENIAL

The first reaction is usually *denial*. Denial serves as a self-protection mechanism. It allows you time to gather your thoughts and to gear up for dealing with the situation at hand. The timing of denial is not preset; that is, everyone does not experience it at the same point. For some women, it may be important to handle the details of scheduling surgery (arranging time off, cleaning up loose ends, arranging for help after surgery) first, then confronting surgery and recovery with seeming bravery and acceptance only to confront denial at a later point in time. Experiencing denial once does not preclude its happening again—you may deal with it many times on the road to acceptance.

ANGER

When you can no longer deny that the hysterectomy is going to happen to you—that this very real situation will have an effect on your life, then you may begin to feel *anger*. You may displace this anger, believing that everything and everybody is in some way responsible for the predicament you now find yourself in. An example of this anger might be, "Why is the medical profession so incompetent? If they really knew what they were doing, they would have found a cure by now and I would not need a hysterectomy."

The anger may also take on a more personal aspect. Instead of blaming outsiders you might begin to blame yourself—for not seeing your gynecologist sooner, or for not demanding more aggressive treatment, or maybe for the lifestyle that you've chosen. Your family and friends will not find it easy to help you with your anger. The very best that they can do is to listen to you and offer comfort and love.

Feeling anger and rage is neither bad nor unhealthy. In fact, it is understandable, given the attitudes that we hold to in this society. Most people assume that if they lead a good and ethical life, eat a fairly decent diet and take care of their bodies, that nothing bad will ever happen to them. Unfortunately, the ugly truth is that taking care of your body (exercise and diet, regular checkups, no smoking, light drinking) certainly will lower the likelihood of certain diseases occurring, but it does not guarantee problem-free health. Your need for a logical explanation for the rhetorical question of "why is this happening?"—to which there is no satisfactory answer—leads to frustration and anger.

BARGAINING

As anger subsides, fear emerges and with it the need to *bargain*. Fear of the unknown may prompt you into bargaining for "one last chance." You need not be of any particular religion to bargain. It seems that people bargain with an interdenominational higher power. Some examples of bargaining might be: "Allow me to get pregnant and I promise I'll have the hysterectomy immediately after the baby is born," or "I promise to have the hysterectomy as soon as I find the right man to marry." Or, "I'll change my lifestyle (work less and nurture more) if you let me keep my reproductive capabilities."

Bargaining is a variation of denial, a mechanism used to postpone the inevitable. The bargain is in effect a prize awarded for good behavior. Bargaining comes about in part because of guilt—guilt that perhaps you were remiss in various areas of your life. Now that you have seen the light, you will make amends and therefore will be spared. Usually, the bargain has a time limit on it (until marriage, pregnancy). And even if the bargain were granted, the bargainer would never be willing to accept those limits and would probably ask for another extension.

Since the bargaining stage is usually very private, friends and family can't help much at this point. Bargaining is a natural response to a situation in which you actually have minimal control. However, understand that while the act of bargaining is interesting and provides some respite from the pressures of dealing with the situation, no matter what you promise to do and no matter how well you do it, you do not have the capacity to change the facts of the situation you're confronted with.

DEPRESSION

During any type of illness, people lose a certain degree of independence and control over their lives. Loss of control stems from the physical and psychological pain of the illness, the type of treatment needed, or the overall effects on the quality of life. *Depression* is often the response to the physiologic withdrawal of estrogen combined with the response of this type of sudden, dramatic loss.

A woman facing a hysterectomy may find it depressing to consider how she will be perceived by her partner sexually, or more important, how she will see herself. Women who have had their ovaries removed may be frightened of all the menopausal symptoms that may await them. The symptoms can be severe, such as hot flashes, night sweats, decreased libido. She may wonder about hormonal therapy and its risks. The fatigue of having undergone major surgery and the slow process of recovery also contribute to depression.

This type of depression may take many forms. You may think wistfully of what might have been; you may be devastated by what this event means for your future, or you may experience numerous other feelings in between. Sadness is a normal response to unpleasant and uncomfortable reality, a healthy part of the total grieving process. However, at some point it can stop being healthy grieving and begin to be unhealthy depression. Family and friends can be most helpful by being patient and understanding. This is not always an easy task for them when you are not proceeding through this process at the rate that they think you should. Be patient with yourself! You have had a great deal to digest and handle, so allow yourself ample time to mourn. Once you have completed this process you begin to rebuild your life.

ACCEPTANCE

It is at this point that you have reached *acceptance*. You will be able to talk about what makes you angry, sad and uncomfortable, but the difference is that you have accepted the diagnosis, the hysterectomy and the ramifications of the surgery. This acceptance comes with the realization that although there is nothing you can do to change the situation, you are now ready to handle it in a responsible way.

Acceptance is often misinterpreted as passive resignation because you have adopted a calmer manner. During this most exciting stage of mourning, you will be setting your course for the future, demonstrating that you are once again in control of your life.

DIFFERENTIATING BETWEEN NORMAL GRIEF AND UNHEALTHY DEPRESSION

Sadness is a normal response to negative events. Such events might include illness, death, loss of employment, marriage (all marriages have their normal ups and downs) and divorce. Depression, on the other hand, is an extreme response to events (positive and negative) due to distorted thoughts about those events. An example of this type of thinking might be: "Because of the hysterectomy, I am worthless as a woman," or "Because of the hysterectomy, I am never going to enjoy sex again." Both examples illustrate valid but greatly distorted concerns (identity questioning and sexuality). Once you eliminate the exaggerated aspects of such thinking and feelings, fears and/or problems become more manageable if not solvable.

Depression can turn into a vicious cycle. You may have difficulty putting an end to it all by yourself, because it is based on a series of interlocking thoughts from which there seems no way out. You may be uncomfortably aware that something is wrong, but feel unable to name it or handle it. It can be useful, if not essential, to seek help from an understanding friend or friends, a woman's self-help hysterectomy group, or an appropriate health care professional—someone who has had experience in talking with posthysterectomy women.

Selecting someone to help you with your mental health is just as important as selecting someone to tend to your physical needs. The following suggestions can be used as a guide for selecting help:

1. Find someone who is able to put your needs and best interests first.
2. Inquire as to whether or not the therapist has any experience in dealing with posthysterectomy women.
3. Inquire about the use of tranquilizers (if tranquilizers are part of

the standard operating practice, perhaps your interests would be better served elsewhere).

4. Ask about the fee schedule. (Most therapists offer a sliding fee scale for clients.)
5. If you are checking out a self-help group, find out who acts as the group's facilitator. (It is useful to know if the facilitator is a lay-person or an experienced counselor. If you are having mild problems, a self-help group with a lay leader is fine, but if you're having more complicated problems you will want the support of a more experienced professional.)

The first step toward recovery from depression is to recognize the problem. The following stories help make clear what sorts of behaviors are normal and which are extreme.

Marie, a forty-two-year-old marketing rep for a medium-size advertising company, had a hysterectomy and oophorectomy six months ago. Returning to work after taking six weeks of leave, she finds it extremely difficult to concentrate. It takes her an inordinate amount of time to accomplish even the smallest task. Her supervisor has noticed that Marie's interpersonal skills have weakened and her slowness is having an impact on the success of several accounts. Marie knows that something is wrong but cannot put her finger on what it is. She doesn't sleep as well as she used to, has no appetite (she has lost fifteen pounds), and she feels isolated from the people she was once close to. As she puts it, "I'm running hard just to keep up a snail's pace."

Marie has some of the key indicators for depression: weight loss, sleep disturbance, inability to concentrate, feelings of isolation. If she were to continue on without the help of a mental health professional, there's a chance that the depression might worsen, making recovery longer and more difficult.

Marie's problems are obvious to all, including herself. Sometimes depression can manifest itself in more subtle ways:

Sally had her hysterectomy four months ago at the age of twenty-five. It was difficult for her to leave the hospital. She had been so seriously ill that she felt nervous about being on her own. Everyone remarked at how quickly she was able to put her life back together. In four months she was able to create enough paintings to take part in a special gallery exhibition. Everything seemed fine to everyone except Sally. She just didn't know how to be happy. She seemed okay most of the time, but had crying spells and occasional problems sleeping. While she seemed to be relating well to her peers and colleagues, she maintained a distance with everyone.

Though Sally seems to be doing well, she is having some problems with depression, albeit a mild to moderate case. Mild or severe depression definitely affects the overall quality of life.

DEPRESSION CHECKLIST

If you are worried about whether or not you are suffering from depression, take a look at the following checklist of warning signals:

Are you having problems sleeping?	yes___	no___
Has your appetite decreased?	yes___	no___
Has your appetite increased?	yes___	no___
Have you lost more than ten pounds?	yes___	no___
Have you gained more than ten pounds?	yes___	no___
Do you feel sad most of the time?	yes___	no___
Do you have problems concentrating?	yes___	no___
Do you have problems making decisions?	yes___	no___
Are you dissatisfied with your life?	yes___	no___
Do you feel guilty most of the time?	yes___	no___
Do you feel discouraged about the future?	yes___	no___
Do you feel that you have failed at life?	yes___	no___
Do you feel that God is punishing you?	yes___	no___
Do you cry more than you used to?	yes___	no___
Do you think of killing yourself?	yes___	no___
Do you hate yourself?	yes___	no___
Do you think that you are unattractive?	yes___	no___
Are you more easily annoyed?	yes___	no___
Have you lost interest in other people?	yes___	no___
Are you uncomfortable around other people?	yes___	no___
Are you disinterested in sex?	yes___	no___

If you answered yes to five or more of these questions, it would be a good idea to contact a therapist.

If you need assistance with your problems, there are mental health professionals who are experienced in dealing with people who suffer from depression as a result of a physical illness. The best way to find such a therapist is to contact the hospital's social services department and ask for a referral. The social services department should have a complete listing of psychiatrists, psychologists and clinical social workers along with a description of their practice and/or area of professional interest. Local chapters of the professional associations for social workers, psychologists and psychiatrists may also be useful in giving information about a potential therapist.

Don't be ashamed to seek help for a problem too big for you to handle alone. Act wisely! It won't really matter very much that your body is healed if your mind is severely troubled—the body and mind work hand-in-hand to promote overall good health.

HOW TO BEGIN TO REBUILD

Now is a good time to take stock of your life. Take a look at the various aspects of it (personal, professional, social, spiritual and recreational), and try to determine what you like about your life and what you don't like and how to go about changing it. There is no need to feel limited by these categories. These are simply examples of areas that may be of importance to you.

The best way to begin assessing your life is to do the following:

Divide a piece of paper into five sections. Give each section a heading (professional, social, etc.)
Write down your achievements in each of the areas.
Write down your weaknesses in each of the areas.
Determine a goal for each category and write it down.

Physical and emotional recovery take time and a commitment from you to work toward getting better. You may become tired and frustrated at times, but the payoff is well worth it.

Surgical Menopause and Hormonal Therapy

Surgical menopause follows the surgical removal of the ovaries, causing a sudden onset of the menopausal symptoms that begin taking place naturally around the age of forty-five. The most common symptoms are:

- hot flashes
- vaginal atrophy
- decreased libido
- mood swings
- osteoporosis

HOT FLASH AND HOT FLUSH

Hot flash and hot flush are terms describing the sudden rushes of warmth felt by a postmenopausal woman. The two terms actually describe two related, but different symptoms. The hot flash refers to the subjective feeling a woman has prior to the physical measurable change—the hot flush.[9] The hot flash precedes the flush by an average time of forty-five seconds. There is little correlation between the intensity of the flash and the amount of measurable change in skin temperature.

The hot flash feels like a sudden rush of warmth. The subsequent flush occurs with redness of the face, neck and upper chest, followed by profuse sweating in the reddened areas for a duration of two to three minutes. Flushing occurs because the body's central thermostat (lo-

57

cated in the brain) is responding to the hot flash. The body begins to compensate by dilatation of the skin blood vessels and by perspiration.

The onset of hot flushes is caused, at least in part, by a sudden drop in estrogen levels after the surgical removal of the ovaries (oophorectomy). The hot flush actually seems to be a physical response to estrogen withdrawal as opposed to having too little estrogen. That is, once the body has adjusted to a different level of estrogen, the flushing episodes should lessen. This adjustment may take from six months to three years.

When you are trying to determine what, if any, medical intervention is appropriate for your menopausal symptoms, it would be useful to keep a log of your flushing episodes. This log should indicate the type of flush (mild, moderate or severe), the duration and the number of episodes each day. In a mild episode the symptoms are barely noticeable. The feeling of warmth associated with little if any perspiration lasts for less than one minute. This type of flash/flush comes and goes with minimal disruption to your activities. The moderate flash/flush episode is warmer, more noticeable and produces perspiration in specific areas of the body for a duration of two to three minutes. This type of flash/flush episode can make you somewhat uncomfortable. You may want to remove a layer or two of clothing to help cool yourself. Your activities are mildly disrupted for the duration of this experience. The severe flash/flush episode feels extremely hot, causing profuse perspiration over the entire body. You will want to remove several layers of clothing, get a cool drink and fan yourself. Severe episodes last longer, cause more distraction and can leave you feeling distressed, frustrated and unable to cope. A sample log page might look like this:

TABLE 2

	Intensity	Duration	Frequency
Monday	severe	3.5 minutes	35 times
Tuesday	severe	3-4 minutes	39 times
Wednesday	severe	3-4 minutes	30 times
Thursday	severe	4 minutes	38 times
Friday	severe	4 minutes	50 times
Saturday	severe	4 minutes	50 times
Sunday	severe	4-5 minutes	60 times

The symptoms illustrated in table 2 represent those of a woman who is in a great amount of discomfort. It would be reasonable and appropriate for this woman to seek out medical advice for help in handling these episodes.

Let's consider what is happening to this woman. Her severe flash/flush episodes occur on the average 120 to 200 minutes per day. This represents approximately 2 to 3.5 hours of her life every day. It's no wonder that women who have moderate to severe symptoms report feeling frustrated and unable to cope. The most convenient and most frequently used method of handling these symptoms is hormonal therapy. The benefits and risks of hormonal treatment will be addressed later in this chapter. For now, let's examine the nonhormonal methods for coping with the hot flash/flush syndrome.

COPING WITH SYMPTOMS

For women who are trying to cope with symptoms in the moderate to severe range, these few tips may make your life more comfortable:

- Wear natural fiber clothing (cotton, linen, wool). If you perspire frequently, you'll feel fresher and more comfortable in a cotton blouse than in a silk or synthetic blend.
- Dress in layers of clothing. Wear a sweater over your blouse on cool days or even a vest. Then when you have a flushing episode, you can take off the vest or cardigan temporarily until your symptoms subside.
- Avoid alcohol, caffeine and sugar as much as possible. These three substances seem to trigger flash/flush episodes. It would be prudent to avoid these substances whenever possible.
- If possible, take a tepid shower when you're feeling uncomfortable. It's a quick way to cool down during a flush.
- If you are taking medications, check with your gynecologist to make certain the medications are not triggering the flush.
- With regard to night sweats, sleep in a cotton or other natural fabric gown, use a cotton blanket or light comforter. Some women have reported sticking one foot out from under the blankets often helps cool down during a "sweat."

- Carry a fan in your purse or briefcase (the hand-operated oriental type is perfect).

These tips will certainly offer a little help. If that help is not enough, perhaps you may want to try other alternatives before considering the use of hormones.

BIOFEEDBACK

Preliminary research in biofeedback training to help control the intensity of the flash/flush episodes has yielded encouraging results.[10]

Biofeedback allows you to monitor your own body functions, such as heart rate, skin temperature, muscle tension, and use that information (feedback) to control those functions.

The idea behind biofeedback is this: If you can successfully raise your skin temperature (using biofeedback techniques) you'll experience slight discomfort or none at all during the flash/flush episode because you will have lessened the extreme difference in body temperature.

While biofeedback plays a valid and useful role in the management of flash/flush episodes, it is not a technique that physicians readily turn to. Most mainstream physicians consider it to be an alternative treatment method with some beneficial results. For more detailed information regarding biofeedback therapy, contact the hospital social worker, your gynecologist, or ask the National Association of Biofeedback Therapists (see Appendix 2 for a complete address) for a list of qualified therapists in your area.

VITAMINS

Some women report that vitamin B-complex and vitamin E have been helpful in combatting hot flashes. Vitamin B-complex aids in the detoxification and elimination of FSH and LH (Follicle Stimulating Hormone and Luteinizing Hormone) by the liver. High FSH and LH levels seem to be linked to frequent hot flashes. Adding supplements of B-complex will not eliminate flashes, although it may help control them. Wheat germ, yogurt, whole grains, brewer's yeast and milk are all good sources of B vitamins.

When women take vitamin E for menopausal discomfort they report that it makes them feel very good in addition to providing relief from hot flashes. They have more energy and a better outlook on life.[11] Increases in FSH and LH production have been related to vitamin E deficiency. The body's requirement for vitamin E increases during periods of stress or extra demands on the reproductive system. The menopausal woman may be deficient in vitamin E, leading to increased FSH production (which is thought to be one cause of hot flashes). It can take up to four weeks for vitamin E to be effective. It is not recommended for use by women with diabetes, hypertension or rheumatic heart disease. Vitamin E can be found in such foods as vegetable oils, wheat germ, soybeans, peanuts and spinach.

A word of caution regarding vitamins—stick to the recommended dose. The idea that if one is good, then two must be better is rubbish. You could possibly permanently damage some vital organs by taking too high a dosage.

Many people use ginseng, an oriental herb, to promote healing. It seems to have a normalizing action on the body and helps in promoting adaptation to heat stress.[12] Although there are no hard data to prove the effectiveness of ginseng on menopausal symptoms, many women report that it has either relieved or eliminated their hot flushes. You can find ginseng extract at health food stores.

IMAGERY
Recent research validates the importance of the mind-body connection in the area of health care.[13] Numerous mental health professionals have discussed the power of the mind and its effect on the body's functioning, and researchers are generating new scientific data to support such claims. With this in mind it might be appropriate to consider the concept of imagery as a method to help not only with hot flash/flush episodes, but with the overall healing process.

Imagery or creative visualization is a method of using your imagination to create a specific scene in your life. Most of us have experienced imagery from time to time. Perhaps another way of describing it would be to call it creative daydreaming. You create a scene from your life, write the dialogue and determine the outcome. In other words, you are in control of the situation. You can use imagery to help achieve many types of goals. For example, you might want to improve your self-esteem level, improve your professional status, or lose weight. Imagery can assist you in successfully achieving that goal. While imagery can help you crystallize and achieve your goals, it is not magic. It is but one of many tools that you may utilize to achieve good health.

The technique is a straightforward one. Simply follow these steps:

1. Go to a place where you will not be disturbed.
2. Sit in a chair or comfortable place.
3. The room should have soft, gentle lighting. Candlelight is good.
4. Begin to focus on your breathing. Slow down your breathing and with each exhalation concentrate on making your body relax to the point that you feel you are afloat.
5. Starting with the tips of your toes and ending with the hair on your head, concentrate first on tensing a part of the body and then relaxing that same part. By the time you reach your hair you will feel light and relaxed.
6. Picture yourself in pleasant surroundings (beach, mountains, tropical paradise, meadow). Make certain to set the entire scene (including smells, sounds, flowers, animals, people). This is your scene, so make it good for yourself.
7. Maintain this scene and picture your relaxed body in this vision for a few minutes.
8. Now picture what the hot flash/flush must look like. Assign it a character. Think of it as being a weak character, one that can and will be overpowered by something much stronger . . . you!
9. Now picture how you are going to combat the flash. Make sure to assign it a strong powerful character, a character that will neutralize and destroy without hesitation the weaker character.
10. Actively visualize the destruction of the force causing the hot flash for a few minutes.
11. Continue to visualize yourself as being in control of your body and capable of decreasing the effect the flash episodes have

on your day-to-day activities. Visualize yourself as a strong
and healthy woman.

12. Begin to focus once again on your breathing and take a few
    deep breaths. When you exhale, imagine that you are expel-
    ling all of the things that prevent you from being in control.

13. At this point the visualization exercise is completed. You may
    open your eyes and resume normal activities. It is useful to
    complete steps 1 through 7 several times a day to help with
    general relaxing. However, when you are having a flash/flush
    episode remember what you have learned about relaxation
    and its effects on your body when under stress. You can then
    implement a quick draw type of imagery by following steps 8
    through 12. Imagery or visualization will not cure or stop hot
    flash/flush episodes, but it can help bring you back into kilter
    after being disoriented, and lessen the overall disruption to
    your life, by giving you better coping skills.

VAGINAL ATROPHY

Vaginal atrophy refers to the thinning of the vaginal walls and the loss of
elasticity. It usually occurs following the removal of the ovaries
(oophorectomy) or natural menopause although women who have had
hysterectomy without removal of the ovaries have reported vaginal
dryness. Atrophy usually occurs when estrogen levels decrease. This
condition can cause burning, itching and painful intercourse, and make
women more susceptible to vaginal and bladder infections.

There are some nonhormonal methods of dealing with this problem:

1. Use a lubricant such as Lubrin vaginal suppositories or K-Y jelly
   during intercourse. Lubrin seems to be the best lubricant
   available because it produces long-lasting lubrication that is
   very similar to what your body used to produce naturally. Both
   are available without a prescription.

2. Vitamin E supplements over an extended period of time have
   been helpful to some women.

3. Doing Kegel exercises on a regular basis (approximately one

hundred to three hundred daily) promotes healing, increases lubrication and improves muscle tone.[14] (Kegel exercises are explained in Chapter 6. Basically, they involve long and short contractions of the muscle which supports and surrounds the sexual organs.)

4. Remain sexually active. Intercourse helps in maintaining the pliability of the vaginal tissue.

DECREASED LIBIDO

Many women who have undergone hysterectomy and oophorectomy report a drop in libido (sexual urge). The loss of hormones from the ovaries, in particular androgen, is the primary cause for loss of libido.

But the desire for sex also depends on the mind and how you feel about yourself and your partner. There are many reasons why a woman fresh from hysterectomy and/or oophorectomy might have difficulties focusing on reestablishing a healthy sex life. She may fear the pain her condition caused during intercourse before the operation; she may feel ugly and disfigured; or she may find that abnormal pelvic tension in the months following the operation makes sex painful. However, with a bit of creative thinking and implementation, a woman can rediscover the joy of a sexually fulfilling relationship. The use of fantasy as well as other sexual exercises for the woman and her partner will be discussed more fully in the chapter on sexual functioning.

MOOD SWINGS

Mood swings are often a psychological effect of surgical menopause. There are several theories about estrogen levels and mood swings. One theory suggests that the autonomic nervous system develops a sensitivity to estrogen and consequently becomes dependent on its balance. Estrogen withdrawal disrupts this balance and this disruption is manifested in the systems controlled by the autonomic nervous system. Symptoms most commonly reported are irritability, anxiety, confusion and depression. While estrogen withdrawal and mood fluctuations are clearly connected, the physical wear and tear of hysterectomy and/or oophorectomy and its psychological ramifications may also contribute to such mood swings.

OSTEOPOROSIS

Osteoporosis (figure 5.1) refers to the loss of bone mass or thinning of the bones. Osteoporosis has been attributed to estrogen decline and withdrawal. Men and women reach peak bone mass by age thirty-five. After age thirty-five either a plateau is maintained or loss of bone mass begins. When women have their ovaries removed, loss of bone mass begins sooner. Because osteoporosis gives no clear warning symptoms, women are usually unaware that they have the disease until after their first fracture. In light of this information the best defense is prevention.

There are two general types of osteoporosis—primary and secondary. Secondary osteoporosis usually occurs as a result of some specific disease or drug (such as bone cancer or steroids). Secondary osteoporosis can occur in men as well as women, and in children as well as adults. Primary osteoporosis, however, usually results from the interaction of several factors—heredity, nutrition, exercise and hormones.

Every bone is composed of two types of bone tissue. Cortical tissue is the solid and dense bone material that surrounds the inner bone. The

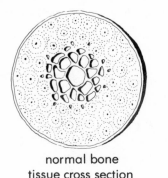
normal bone
tissue cross section

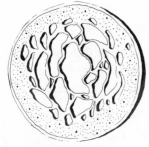
osteoporotic bone
tissue cross section

Figure 5.1   Osteoporosis

inner portion, trabecular bone, is more porous and therefore more easily affected by bone mass loss. When osteoporosis occurs, the trabecular bone becomes more porous than normal and its outside protective bone cover becomes thinner, making women more susceptible to fractures and breaks.

WHO'S AT RISK?
Women at the highest risk of developing osteoporosis are:

- women who experience menopause or oophorectomy at an early age;
- women with a family history of osteoporosis;
- Caucasian women are more at risk than black women;
- women who have had any of the following disorders: kidney disease, diabetes, rheumatoid arthritis and hyperthyroidism;
- thin or slender women;
- women who eat a poor, unbalanced diet;
- women who lead a sedentary lifestyle;
- women who have a heavy intake of tobacco, caffeine, protein or alcohol;
- women who have experienced one or more osteoporotic fractures.

BE AWARE OF THE WARNING SIGNS
Early detection of this condition seems to be quite elusive to medical science. Some warning signs that you should report immediately to your physician are:

- loose or transparent skin;
- symptoms of gum disease (excessive bleeding, swelling, etc.);
- signs of shrinking or decreased height.

One or more of these symptoms coupled with any of the ten risk factors is sufficient reason to seek a diagnosis from your physician. Since the muscular-skeletal area is the medical domain of the orthopedist, it will be necessary to ask your gynecologist for a referral.

Many tests exist which can confirm a diagnosis of osteoporosis, and assess its severity. But there are virtually no noninvasive tests to identify a woman's predisposition to developing osteoporosis.

If you want more extensive information about osteoporosis, the latest detection methods, etc. contact your local menopause care center. There is also an excellent book: *Stand Tall! The Informed Woman's Guide to Osteoporosis* by Morris Notelovitz, M.D., Ph.D., and Marsha Ware, Triad, 1982.

WHAT YOU CAN DO TO HELP PREVENT OSTEOPOROSIS

Follow a sound nutritional program. Women need between 1200 and 1500 mg of elemental calcium per day. Because women tend to be calorie-conscious they usually avoid the foods that are high in calcium (milk, cheese, and nuts). To achieve daily requirements it may be necessary to use calcium supplements. Several over-the-counter supplements are:

Os-Cal-500 tablets 1250 mg CaCO3 (500 mg elemental calcium)
Calcium Carbonate 650 mg CaCO3 (250 mg calcium)
Calcium gluconate 1000 mg CaGluc (100 mg calcium)
One-a-day plus minerals (100 mg calcium)

All calcium supplements are not the same. It is important to determine the number of tablets necessary to achieve the daily requirements. Take calcium tablets twice daily and never take more calcium than is recommended. (See Table 6 at the end of the chapter for a list of foods and the calcium mg assigned to each.)

Vitamin D, important and essential for bone metabolism, also stimulates bone growth. The recommended dose of vitamin D is 400 mg per day. A few foods are high in vitamin D. Most milk is fortified with 100 IU (international units) of vitamin D per cup. Excess vitamin D can be toxic, so be certain not to exceed the recommended dose.

Limit and maintain your protein intake at 44 grams daily. A high-protein diet requires more calcium to process it, which adds to your overall bone loss.

Avoid or restrict your use of caffeine, cigarettes, alcohol and salt.

Women who smoke, drink excessive alcohol and/or caffeinated beverages and use large amounts of salt lose more calcium than women who avoid tobacco, caffeine, alcohol and salt.

Develop and maintain a regular exercise program. Thirty to sixty minutes of weight-bearing exercise such as walking, cycling, and dancing performed three to five times per week is adequate. Regular exercise stimulates bone formation; however, excessive amounts of exercise can be damaging and increase the amount of bone loss.

HORMONAL THERAPY

Hormonal replacement therapy (HRT) is the use of hormones (estrogens and/or progesterones) to control or prevent symptoms of estrogen deficiency such as hot flashes, vaginal atrophy and osteoporosis.

Before deciding to start hormonal therapy, weigh the risks carefully. For example, if you had your surgery because of an estrogen-dependent disease, it is crucial to weigh your need for symptom control over the possibility that the hormone treatments will bring back your disease. Other physiological conditions may signal that hormonal therapy is not appropriate for you. The following table lists medical problems that should be monitored during hormonal therapy and medical problems that prohibit hormonal therapy:

TABLE 3

Conditions to Be Monitored	Conditions Prohibiting HRT
Family history of Breast Cancer	Breast Cancer
Fibrocystic Breast Condition	Uterine Cancer
Liver Disease	History of Heart Attack
Gall Bladder Disease	History of Stroke
Diabetes	Thrombosis
Phlebitis	Undiagnosed vaginal bleeding
Gross Obesity	
High Blood Pressure	
Heavy Smoking	
Migraine	

If you have one or more medical conditions but still think that HRT would be beneficial, you might discuss with your physician the possibility of reducing some of the risk factors. For example, if you are a heavy smoker and overweight, you might consider eliminating smoking altogether and reducing your caloric intake. Excess weight, smoking and lack of exercise are proven hazards to your overall health, so if you can change these habits by all means do so.

Before beginning any regimen of hormone replacement therapy, your gynecologist or endocrinologist should evaluate your health status. A proper evaluation will include:

> breast exam (including mammography)
> Pap smear
> complete physical exam
> complete blood analysis

This information gives your physician a baseline for you to determine which dosage level is best, and allows him/her to spot any abnormalities as a result of HRT.

Contact your physician if you notice any major changes in your health patterns. Otherwise, make your first follow-up visit at one month and thereafter semiannually. If you adhere to this suggested schedule, either you or your physician should be able to detect any abnormalities before they get out of control.

ESTROGEN REPLACEMENT THERAPY

Estrogen is rarely given by itself these days, although there are some gynecologists who prescribe it alone to combat menopausal symptoms. Estrogen is safest and most effective when taken in combination with progesterone to control menopausal symptoms. Since estrogen has raised numerous questions with regard to its causal relationship with breast cancer, liver disorder, and other undesirable side effects, let's take a look at the risks, benefits and methods of estrogen administration.

The most frequently prescribed estrogen is taken orally, in the form of a pill. There are two types of estrogen: natural and synthetic. Oral preparations of estrogens must be processed and absorbed through the liver. Research data support the claims that natural estrogens are better absorbed (for the most part) than the synthetic estrogens. Premarin, a brand of natural estrogen, contains approximately 30 percent horse estrogen. The presence of the horse estrogen may account for the slight adverse effect on liver functions.

See table 4 for a chart identifying natural and synthetic estrogens.

TABLE 4

Estrogens	Trade Name	Manufacturer
Natural	Premarin	Ayerst
	Ogen	Abbott
	Estrace	Mead-Johnson
	Menrium (estrogen plus Librium, a tranquilizer)	Roche
Synthetic	Estinyl (estrogen used in birth control)	Schering
	Estrovis	Parke-Davis

It is best to approach estrogens with caution. Most gynecologists prefer to start women on the lowest dose of natural estrogen available (the lowest dose available is 0.3 mg and the highest is 3.0 mg). If the symptoms are not kept at bay with the absolute lowest level, then the dosage level would very gradually be increased to the next level. Be careful to report your symptoms accurately: Keep a log of the intensity and frequency of your symptoms. While it is important to get relief from menopausal symptoms, it is equally important not to use more estrogen than is absolutely necessary.

In addition to estrogens in pill form, you can have *injections, subcutaneous implants, Band-aid type patches, vaginal rings,* and *estrogen creams.* These alternative methods of estrogen delivery are currently being used by less than 5 percent of menopausal women. One reason so few women use these methods is because some of them are still experimental; to use them, you must agree to take part in a research study. If you decide to do so, you will be advised of the risks and side effects and required to sign an Informed Consent document. More physicians will suggest and implement these alternative forms once their effectiveness has been proven. These parenteral (medication that is not processed through the intestines), nonoral methods of estrogen administration are often more desirable because the estrogen is absorbed directly into the bloodstream and not processed through the stomach, liver and intestines.

Intramuscular injections are usually given on a three to six week schedule. One drawback of the intramuscular injection is that the dosage of estrogen is not easily controlled.

Subcutaneous implants are very effective in arresting menopausal symptoms. The implant can be inserted in your gynecologist's office under local anesthesia. A small incision is made in the groin and the implant is inserted through a tube. The tube is later removed and the pellet is pushed into the fat under the skin. A single stitch closes the opening, so that scarring will be minimal for this procedure. The implant remains effective for approximately one year in most women. However, a new implant can be inserted if the symptoms should recur earlier than one year. The major drawback to this type of treatment is that because the implant is difficult to find it is practically impossible to remove should you have negative side effects.

Some women who have difficulties in processing oral estrogens are using *vaginal rings,* which seem to provide effective dosages of estrogen over a three-month period of time. The ring does not interfere with sexual intercourse because it can be removed during intercourse and replaced afterward. Vaginal discharge seems to be one of the side effects of this type of estrogen administration.

The estrogen patch delivers the hormone continuously through the skin in very small amounts at a controlled rate. The patch must be changed twice a week. It can be worn conveniently on the upper arm or torso.

Estrogen creams can be applied to the lower abdomen and directly into the vagina. The dosage level has to be repeated every twenty-four hours to remain effective. Long term use of vaginal estrogen has the same negative effects as oral estrogen.

COMBINED ESTROGEN AND PROGESTERONE THERAPY

The addition of progesterone to HRT has neutralized many of the negative side effects estrogen seemed to produce. Progesterone is usually given for ten days each month frequently at the end of the cycle. (For example: A woman takes only 0.625 mg of oral estrogen on day 1 through day 13; on day 14, she begins taking 10 mg of progesterone in addition to the estrogen; and on day 20 she stops all hormones for the next 7 days and then repeats the entire cycle again.)

Information about progesterone is not as comprehensive as it is for estrogen. However, it has been suggested that the estrogen-progesterone combination may cause heart disease, stroke, weight gain and depression. It is very difficult to assess which side effects are attributable to the interaction of progesterone and estrogen and which to progesterone alone. There are several synthetic and only one natural progesterone. The natural progesterone in oil is available in injection and suppository form. Table 5 offers a list of synthetic progesterones.

TABLE 5

Progestins	Trade Name	Manufacturer
Synthetic	Provera	Upjohn
	Megace	Mead-Johnson
	Norlutin	Warner-Lambert

Several problems and conditions have been linked with hormone replacement therapy—breast cancer and migraine are just two examples. Most physicians will rely very strongly on your family breast history as well as your own breast conditions in assessing the value of hormone therapy for you. If you have a history of fibrocystic breast condition and a strong family history of breast cancer, your physician should administer a very low dosage of estrogen and progesterone to handle the symptoms. He/she should also watch your breasts very closely to observe and address any changes.

With respect to HRT and migraine, neurologists have found that the problem relates to the cyclical nature of the HRT administration. What some neurologists suggest is that a woman be placed on the lowest dosages possible for a continuous period of time. Instead of the twenty-one day cycle, HRT would be administered over an extended period with no breaks. It seems that the problem of migraine arises as a direct result of hormonal fluctuation, so if the hormonal levels remain constant the woman won't be bothered by as many migraine headaches.[15]

Hormonal replacement therapy is very tricky. It is crucial to work closely and carefully with your physician so that dosage levels can be carefully adjusted for the maximum amount of relief with the minimal amount of negative side effects.

ALTERNATIVE DRUGS

If it is impossible for you to take estrogens without risking serious consequences, then the following drugs may be of interest to you:

Bellergal (a drug containing a sedative and sympathetic and para-sympathetic nervous system inhibitors) has been given for many years to help relieve hot flash/flush episodes. It operates on the premise that flashes and flushes occur because of the overactivity of the sympathetic and parasympathetic nervous systems. Bellergal corrects the imbalance and thereby decreases the flashing episodes.

Clonidine is often used in treating hypertensive individuals, but is currently being considered as treatment for menopausal woman. Several physicians investigating the drug report that women who take it seem to respond favorably. The frequency, duration and intensity of the flash/flush episodes seemed to be reduced markedly with a small dosage level. The common side effects of Clonidine are dry mouth and sleepiness; less common side effects are: constipation, dizziness, headache and fatigue. Although this drug seems to address the problem of flashing/flushing, there are few data to suggest that it has any effect on osteoporosis or vaginal atrophy.[16]

TABLE 6

CALCIUM, PHOSPHORUS, AND CALCIUM-TO-PHOSPHORUS RATIO OF COMMON FOODS

	Cal (mg)	Phos (mg)	Ratio Ca:P
American cheese, 1 slice	188	208	1:1.1
Apple pie, average slice	9	29	1:2.9
Bacon, cooked, 2 thin slices	1	22	1:22.0
Beans, green, canned, 1 cup	81	50	1:0.6
Beef liver, fried, 1 slice	9	405	1:45.0
Beef noodle soup, canned, 1 cup	7	48	1:6.9
Biscuit mix made with milk, 1 biscuit	19	65	1:3.4
Bologna, 1 slice	1	17	1:17.0
Bran flakes with raisins, 1 cup	28	146	1:5.2
Broccoli (frozen), boiled, 1 cup	100	104	1:1.0
Cauliflower (frozen), boiled, 1 cup	31	68	1:2.2
Cheddar cheese, 1 slice	158	100	1:0.6
Cherry pie, average slice	17	30	1:1.8
Chicken, fried, 1 drumstick	6	89	1:14.8

	Cal (mg)	Phos (mg)	Ratio Ca:P
Chicken chow mein without noodles, homemade, 1 cup	58	293	1:5.1
Chicken noodle soup, canned, 1 cup	10	36	1:3.6
Chili con carne with beans, canned, 1 cup	82	321	1:3.9
Chocolate chip cookies, 4 homemade	14	40	1:2.9
Chocolate devil's food cake, without icing, 1 cupcake	24	45	1:1.9
Coffee, instant, 1 cup	4	7	1:1.8
Corn-on-the-cob, cooked, 1 ear	2	69	1:34.5
Cottage cheese, large curd, 1 cup	212	342	1:1.16
Danish pastry (plain), 1 piece	21	46	1:2.2
Egg, fried, 1 large	28	102	1:3.6
Flounder fillet, baked with butter	23	344	1:15.0
Frankfurter	4	76	1:19.0
French fries, 10 strips	12	87	1:7.3
Ground beef, cooked, 3 ounces	10	196	1:19.6
Ham, baked, 3 ounces	9	201	1:22.3
Hard roll	24	46	1:1.9
Ice-cream, plain, soft-serve, 1 cup	253	199	1:0.8
Lamb chops, broiled, 6 9-ounce chops	24	429	1:17.9
Lettuce, shredded, 1 cup	19	14	1:0.7
Lobster Newburg, 1 cup	218	480	1:2.2
Mashed potatoes, with milk, 1 cup	50	103	1:2.1
Milk, whole, 1 cup	288	227	1:2.8
Minestrone soup, canned, 1 cup	37	59	1:1.6
Oatmeal, cooked, 1 cup	22	137	1:6.2
Orange juice, frozen, 6 ounces	19	32	1:1.7
Peanut butter, 1 tablespoon	9	61	1:6.8
Peanuts, roasted, salted	21	114	1:5.4
Peas (frozen), boiled, 1 cup	30	138	1:4.6
Popcorn, with oil and salt	1	19	1:19.0
Pork and Beans, canned, 1 cup	138	235	1:1.7
Pork chops, broiled, 8 2-ounce chops	28	624	1:22.3
Potato chips, 10 chips	8	28	1:3.5
Pretzels, 10 3-ring pretzels	7	39	1:5.6
Puffed rice cereal	3	13	1:4.7
Pumpkin pie, average slice	58	79	1:1.4
Rice, white, cooked, 1 cup	21	57	1:2.7
Rye bread, 1 slice	19	37	1:1.9
Saltines, 10 crackers	6	26	1:4.3
Sesame seeds, hulled, 1 tablespoon	9	47	1:5.2
Shrimp, french fried, 1 ounce	20	54	1:2.7
Spaghetti, homemade, with tomato sauce, meatballs, Parmesan cheese	124	236	1:1.9
Spinach, canned, 1 cup	242	53	1:0.2

	Cal (mg)	Phos (mg)	Ratio Ca:P
T-Bone steak, cooked, yield from 1 pound raw	24	490	1:20.4
Tomato, 1 average	24	49	1:2.0
Tomato soup, canned, 1 cup	15	34	1:2.3
Tuna, canned, 1 cup	13	374	1:28.8
Vegetable beef soup, canned, 1 cup	12	49	1:4.1
White bread, enriched, 1 slice	24	27	1:1.1
Winter squash, baked, 1 cup	57	98	1:1.7

Sexual Functioning

Healthy, satisfying sexual relationships are not easily achieved even when you are in peak physical and psychological condition. Contrary to popular belief, sex is not a basic instinct, but rather a highly developed and learned skill. Very few people feel complacent about how they perform and respond sexually. When you add to that insecurity the trauma of a gynecological disease, the pain that may have been associated with the disease and the psychological havoc wrought by a hysterectomy, you have a woman and her partner approaching sexual intercourse as if it were a mine field.

Sexual functioning after hysterectomy is one of the areas about which women are most poorly informed. The misinformation is not intentional. In part it results from inaccurate reporting to doctors. Because sexuality is such a personal issue, women are often embarrassed and/or uncomfortable discussing sexual problems with their gynecologists. Many gynecologists are poorly trained when it comes to sexuality and therefore find it difficult to counsel women. But little by little, as women begin sharing information among themselves and passing that information on to their gynecologists and therapists, the situation is improving.

Advice must be tailored to each individual's age and problem. When a twenty-nine-year-old woman has a hysterectomy and oophorectomy because of a severe case of endometriosis (see chapter 1 for a description of the disease), her sexual experience could be positive if the surgery frees her from the severe pain and discomfort after months of agony. On the other hand, her experience could be negative if she associated painful sexual intercourse before surgery with possible painful intercourse after surgery. Other issues that figure in sexual adjustment after hysterectomy are:

- physiological changes brought by surgery
- level of self-esteem before and after surgery
- willingness to work at attaining sexual fulfillment (perhaps with some alteration)
- the effect of hysterectomy on your partner

It is not easy to confront and deal with these issues, but when you address and resolve them one by one, you will be able to enjoy a satisfying sexual relationship once again.

PHYSICAL CHANGES

Although sexual arousal begins primarily in the mind, the body has to be capable of functioning properly in order to achieve pleasure. Some physiological changes following hysterectomy which might make achieving sexual pleasure for all women (straight and lesbian) more challenging are:

shortened length of the vaginal canal
poor vaginal muscle tone
absence of uterine contractions which can mean weaker orgasms
vaginal dryness (occurs in women who have their ovaries removed)
loss of desire (occurs in women who have their ovaries removed)

In radical hysterectomy, approximately one-third of the upper vaginal canal is removed, decreasing the overall length of the vaginal canal. This shortened length does not create problems for most women because the vaginal canal is somewhat elastic, and with time, patience and sufficient lubrication, pleasurable sexual intercourse can be achieved in a reasonably short period of time.

HOW TO COPE WITH THE PHYSICAL CHANGES

If you and your partner experience some difficulties with painful intercourse because of the decreased length, do not be discouraged. You can help stretch the vagina in several ways:

> Use your fingers (two work best) or a dildo to help stretch the vaginal canal. It is often easier for women to get over their fears about penetration if they first do a bit of self-exploration.

> Make love frequently with ample lubrication, allowing the vaginal canal to gradually stretch. Do not use force or roughness.

> Test out different positions for lovemaking. Since there is a problem with length, you will want to find positions that give you control over the depth of penetration. Examples of such positions are: woman on top—in this position you are not only able to control the depth of penetration, but you also increase the amount of clitoral stimulation; lying face to face, side by side—once again you can more easily control the depth of penetration in this position and manual stimulation is less difficult; if you choose the man on top position, you can still control the depth of penetration by moving your legs closer together. Other positions may be more comfortable for you, so experiment until you find a position that is right for you and your partner.

> If after trying the above suggestions you are still having great difficulty, perhaps you need to be evaluated by your gynecologist and/or sex therapist. He/she may suggest the use of vaginal dilators. Vaginal dilators are soft plastic forms inserted into the vagina and left in place for several minutes daily. They gradually and painlessly stretch the vaginal canal.

KEGEL EXERCISES

Poor vaginal and pelvic muscle tone also hinder good sexual functioning. However, with proper exercise not only will the muscle tone improve, but you will promote overall healing and heighten your capability for sexual pleasure. Kegel exercises can do all this for you.

Kegel exercises were developed originally to help women suffering from urinary stress incontinence (a condition in which small amounts of urine are released if a woman coughs, sneezes, jumps or has an orgasm). The exercises work on the pubococcygeal muscle (also known as the PC muscle), which cradles or supports the pelvic organs. In order to determine if you are using the correct muscle, urinate and then contract the muscle that allows you to interrupt the flow of urine. If you can successfully interrupt the flow of urine, then you have found the PC muscle.

You can do a number of different types of Kegel exercises. Some examples are:

Tense-Relax Exercise—Tense or tighten the PC muscle for 2 to 3 seconds and then release that same muscle for 2 to 3 seconds. You should repeat this exercise 10 times at least 3 times daily.

Rapid Tense-Relax—Tense or tighten, then release the PC muscle in rapid succession; that is, you would not hold the muscle for any period of time. Repeat this exercise combination for 10 complete sets at least twice daily.

Gradual Tense-Gradual Relax—Gradually tense the muscles of the vaginal canal beginning at the opening and concluding with the cervix. It will help if you tense the muscles to the count of 10, making sure to distribute the tensing equally over the 10 counts. When you relax those same muscles, begin the relaxation process at the cervix and end at the opening of the vagina. Be sure to distribute the relaxation over the 10 counts. What tends to happen is that women are sometimes unable to completely relinquish all of the tension, so really concentrate on letting go. Repeat this exercise combination at least 3 times daily with a minimum of 10 sets of repetitions.

Tense and Hold and Relax—Tense the PC muscle and hold for a count of 10; then relax the PC muscle over a count of 10. Again, women who have had pelvic trauma (pelvic inflammatory disease, endometriosis, fibroids, cancer) tend to hold tension in their pelvis. It is very difficult for women with these types of experiences to learn to relax those muscles. After all, for many months they have been guarding or tensing the pelvic area because of pain. Now that the pain is theoretically over it is difficult to unlearn those habits. Repeat this exercise in combination 3 times daily with 10 sets of repetitions.

Bear Down and Relax—This exercise involves bearing down, much as you would do during a bowel movement, except you will want to use your vaginal muscles more than your anal ones. As you bear down, imagine that there is something in the vaginal canal that you want to push out. Hold the bearing down portion of this exercise for 3 or 4 seconds and then relax for 3 or 4 seconds.

Each portion of the exercises is important. It will be great if through these exercises you can improve your muscle tone and sexual responsiveness. However, if you have difficulty letting go of the tension you will not be getting the full benefit of the exercise. Tense muscles do not receive the proper blood flow and prohibit proper healing. So, relax.

At first, start out doing each of these exercise combinations ten times at three different times of day. As you feel yourself progress you may want to increase each exercise combination to twenty times at three different times a day.

You might wonder about the side effects of such exercises. Initially you might notice mild discomfort or tension in the pelvic region. If this happens, reduce the number of Kegels you do daily. Whatever happens, don't stop the exercises. The other side effect that some women have mentioned is that while doing the exercises they become sexually aroused. If this should happen to you please do not be alarmed. It is normal to have this sensation. These exercises increase the flow of blood to the pelvic region in much the same way that sexual stimulation does. Don't be alarmed by the arousal you feel. Simply enjoy it and consider it an unexpected benefit.

VAGINAL MYOGRAPH

If after doing the exercises faithfully over a period of a month or so you still don't notice any significant change, perhaps it would be in your best interest to go to a biofeedback therapist. I suggest such a professional because she (most women will be more comfortable with a female therapist in this situation) can accurately measure vaginal tension and strength with a vaginal myograph (or perinometer see figure 6.1), a spoollike soft plastic device shaped like a dumbbell. When inserted vaginally it can provide both therapist and client with information about PC muscle activity. The vaginal myograph is used in conjunction with the regular EMG (electromyographic) biofeedback device.

The vaginal myograph is inserted into the vaginal canal much like a tampon. It fits snugly but comfortably so it does not need to be held in place. The sensors are strategically placed on the myograph measure and record the amount of tension and the level of relaxation in the PC muscle. With the help of a competent therapist you will be able to identify the amount of pelvic tension held normally, the quality of your PC muscle tone, and how able you are to relax those muscles. You will in essence be establishing a starting point or baseline for yourself in assessing your progress. With the help and guidance of your therapist you will be able to identify your problems, zero in on the appropriate exercises and witness the improvements physically and quantitatively.

You probably think that in essence this vaginal myograph is a good idea, but are wondering about the rather personal nature of the device and how it is handled without embarrassment or loss of dignity. Most sex therapists understand the delicate nature of this exercise and

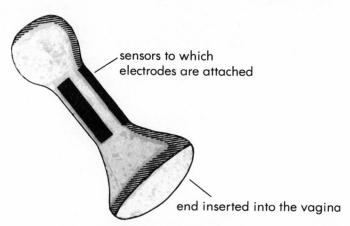

sensors to which electrodes are attached

end inserted into the vagina

Figure 6.1   Vaginal Perinometer
The vaginal perinometer is used in conjunction with biofeedback. It is used to measure muscle tension and tone. The large end of the perinometer is inserted into the vaginal canal.

endeavor to make the client comfortable. At your first visit the therapist will take a history. She will ask questions regarding the onset of your period, surgical history (how many operations and what for), history of venereal disease, history of pelvic trauma (automobile accidents in which pelvis was traumatized, rape and/or incest) and other questions related to your sexual history. She will explain vaginal myograph in great detail, what it is used for, how it can help you, and so forth. At this visit you will also have an opportunity to touch and feel the vaginal myograph. This is the time to ask questions.

Remember, there are no truly stupid questions. If something is making you uncomfortable, speak up and discuss it with your therapist. Chances are that she has answered similar questions before and will not think less of you for asking. Once you understand what is going to happen, the therapist will instruct you as to how to insert the myograph. She will leave the room so that you may maintain maximum privacy and dignity. (It is probably best to wear a skirt or dress to these sessions because you only have to remove your underwear to insert the myograph and can adjust your clothing accordingly.) The therapist will return to your room and begin the session. She will give you instructions such as: tense and hold for ten seconds, tense and hold as long as you can. The first stage of the evaluation may take twenty to thirty minutes. The therapist will then instruct you how to take out the myograph and leave the room. When she returns she will discuss the results of the test and tell you what you need to work on. She will probably send you home with home work (specific Kegel exercises to help you achieve better muscle tone). Work with this type of therapist is usually short term in duration.

While the Kegel exercises and vaginal myograph can help with problems of muscle tone, vaginal dryness (at least to some extent) and decreased length of the vaginal canal, the loss of libido or sexual drive is a separate issue.

FANTASY

Loss of libido often occurs when the ovaries are removed (oophorectomy). It does not happen to every woman, but it occurs with enough regularity to suggest that it is not triggered by some emotional disorder, but rather as a direct result of rapid decrease of estrogen.

If you have difficulties becoming aroused, all is not lost. You will simply have to put more effort into achieving a state of arousal. You can increase your ability to be aroused in several ways. The quickest way—and the most fun—is to experiment with fantasy. Fantasy involves using a pleasant scenario or experience to help you achieve an aroused state. Most people have entertained one or more fantasies in their lifetimes. How simple or complex these fantasies are depends on each person. To help yourself get started thinking about fantasy, let your mind wander to the most pleasant surroundings, with the most interesting and arousing (for you) partner. You don't have to stop with one fantasy, but rather let your mind explore numerous possibilities. Reading erotic books and magazines, and looking at videos can also be sexually exciting.

Many women who have difficulty with spontaneous sexual arousal report that fantasy allows them to get "jump started." They say that by using an erotic illusion or fantasy to enhance their arousal at the beginning of lovemaking they are better able to get into the spirit of the encounter and enjoy the experience. Having a hysterectomy and oophorectomy does not mean that you will be denied satisfying sexual encounters. But it does mean that enjoyable sexual encounters may be more challenging to achieve.

SEXUAL SELF-ESTEEM

In order to know how much work you will need to do and in which areas, it is useful to get an accurate handle on your sexual self-esteem. This assessment is best done in five stages:

> Try to make an estimate of your sexual self-esteem one year prior to the onset of any symptoms of your disease or disorder.
> Make an estimate of your sexual self-esteem two months following surgery.
> Using past and current information regarding your sexual self-esteem, set goals for yourself.
> Try to estimate the effects your hysterectomy has had on your partner.

Determine the level of commitment that you and your partner have toward achieving mutually satisfying sexual relations

Determining your sexual self-esteem level need not be a complicated task. You'll want to know how you feel about yourself as a sexual being. The following quiz will help you get an idea.

1. How satisfied are you with your sex life?
   a) very satisfied
   b) satisfied
   c) dissatisfied
2. How frequently do you make love?
   a) three or more times each week
   b) once or twice each week
   c) once or twice each month
   d) several times yearly
   e) not at all at this time
3. Are you satisfied with the frequency of lovemaking?
   a) yes
   b) no
4. What feelings do you have when you see your nude body?
   a) I like my body and see myself as a sensual person
   b) there are things I'd like to change about my body, but I do feel I am a sensual person
   c) I have an average body with minimal sensuality
   d) I don't like my body and I am not sensual
   e) I am repulsed by my body
5. Who initiates sexual encounters?
   a) you
   b) your partner
6. How frequently do you reach orgasm?
   a) regularly
   b) sometimes
   c) never
7. Is oral sex part of your sex life?
   a) yes
   b) no

8. Is masturbation part of your sex life?
   a) yes
   b) no
9. Is anal intercourse part of your sex life?
   a) yes
   b) no
10. Is sex easily discussed with your partner?
    a) yes
    b) no
11. Are you satisfied with the quality of your sex life?
    a) yes
    b) no

These questions should be answered, in addition to the above questions, two months following surgery:

12. Do you experience any fear when you think about having intercourse?
    a) yes
    b) no
13. What makes you feel this way?
    a) fear that intercourse will cause pain
    b) fear that the disease or disorder will recur
    c) regret that you are no longer able to conceive
    d) fear that you will be unable to reach orgasm
    e) other (please specify)
14. If the frequency of lovemaking has decreased do you think it is because
    a) you feel unappealing to your partner
    b) you feel unappealing to yourself
    c) making love is painful
    d) other (please specify)
15. What would make your sex life more satisfying and enjoyable? (please list everything)

SCORING

There are no correct or incorrect answers to the above questions. The objective of this questionnaire is to provide yourself and your partner with information that will help you understand what things you have to work on. To help make this point clear, read the explanations for each response.

ANSWERS

Question 1

a) If you are very satisfied with your current sex life, the only suggestion to be made is to continue with the level of communication in order to ensure continued satisfaction.

b) If you are satisfied with your sex life take it as a good beginning. Try to identify what keeps your encounters from being better. Once identified it will be easier to address them.

c) If you are dissatisfied with your sex life, don't despair. Once problems are identified and addressed, perhaps you may begin to work on them together or with the help of a reputable sex therapist.

Question 2

a), b), c) Frequency of lovemaking is very personal in that a couple has to come to terms with what is comfortable and satisfying for them. Frequency of sex is often correlated to career, family and physical demands. At this level of frequency there is no reason to feel uncomfortable.

d), e) This level of infrequency suggests that there are problems with normal sexual functioning. The first step is to consult with your physician to ascertain the nature of the problem; next, set goals for yourself; and finally, if necessary, get help from a qualified, reputable sex therapist.

Question 3

a) If your answer is yes and your partner's answer is yes, then you are in good shape. However, if your partner doesn't agree, then the two of you can discuss and reach a compromise.

b) If your answer is no, identify why and set a course for yourself to achieve a level of frequency that is comfortable for you and your partner.

Question 4

a), b) It is important to like your body and yourself—self-love helps us to feel beautiful, wanted and needed. The ability to see yourself as a desirable person helps you to relate to your partner in a more sensual way.

c) There is nothing wrong with being average looking. Too often women are sold a bill of goods with regard to looks and body image. It might be helpful for you to make a list of the things about yourself that you like and a list of things that others have complimented you on. Next, focus on how you feel when complimented about those positive attributes. Savor and bask in that feeling—this is the beginning of feeling good about yourself and feeling sensual.

d), e) If you don't like your body or are repulsed by it, perhaps you need to take a good look at yourself. You may want to shed some weight, try out a more flattering hairstyle, or update your wardrobe. Often cosmetic changes can act as the catalyst for overall internal change. There is always hope for change!

Question 5

a), b) It really doesn't matter which person initiates sexual encounters, there is no right or wrong person to initiate it. However, you or your partner should feel comfortable in initiating sex without the fear of feeling inappropriate.

Question 6

a), b) Some women are better able to achieve orgasm than others. The important thing to remember is that sex is supposed to be a pleasurable experience, so have fun and try not to make having an orgasm the deciding factor for whether or not it is pleasurable.

c) Some women have extreme difficulty in achieving orgasm. Sex therapists have reported that women are more orgasmic after routinely doing the Kegel exercises. There are any number of reasons why a woman has difficulty in achieving orgasm. Get some professional help in sorting this out and the results may be quite favorable.

Question 7

a), b) Oral sex is really a matter of preference for both partners. However, if a couple is experiencing some sexual dysfunction problems, sometimes alternative methods of lovemaking can be explored. Something that may have been uncomfortable for the two of you in the past may be appealing now.

Question 8

a), b) Masturbation is often a way to relieve sexual tension, and also a way to help increase your ability for sexual pleasure. If masturbation is not something you or your partner feel comfortable with, don't force it.

Question 9

a), b) Anal intercourse is something that each partner should agree to before the encounter. Many couples find this alternative method of lovemaking quite satisfying and enjoyable. However, if you and your partner would prefer not to engage in anal intercourse, that's fine too.

Question 10

a) If you and your partner can easily discuss sex, that is an excellent starting point. Whenever there is a sexual misunderstanding or problem, you will be able to confront it with some immediacy and begin to correct or alter the situation.

b) If sex is not a subject that you and your partner can easily discuss, this is your cue to find out what is preventing you from discussing your sex life together. Many people are defensive about their performance (the quality, technique and frequency). If somehow you can remove placing blame and assigning guilt from the discussion, dialogue can begin in a safe setting.

Question 11

a), b) Satisfaction with your sex life today does not assure satisfaction tomorrow and the converse is true. Sex is a learned skill as opposed to an innate trait. With that in mind all people should work toward mutually satisfying sex for the duration of the relationship.

Questions 12, 13, 14 & 15

These questions are to help you get a handle on any specific problems that you may be having following surgery. As stated earlier in this chapter, knowing what the problems are is an important first step toward finding the solution.

Now that you have some information regarding your sexual self-esteem one year prior to your surgery and two months following your surgery, you are in position to set some realistic goals. Be careful not to place too many demands on yourself. Start with one or two goals, but make certain that these are simple enough to be achieved. Once you have achieved some success you will be able to set additional goals. Your level of commitment toward achieving a more satisfying sex life will affect the amount of progress you are able to make. In the meantime, try to have fun and enjoy this sexual rediscovery process.

Hysterectomy tends to take its physical and emotional toll on both partners in a relationship. Consequently, it is in both partners' best interest to vent their feelings about what effect this surgery has had on them. Many women fear that their femininity has been permanently compromised, that they will become old and unattractive, and that depression is all standard fare following this surgery. Some men feel uncomfortable making love to a woman who no longer has the capacity to conceive. It is important to note that this is dysfunctional thinking on their part. Some partners are concerned about catching the disease that made the hysterectomy necessary or perhaps causing the disease to recur. And then there are the men who remember the pain that sexual intercourse caused prior to surgery and who fear that their penises are still instruments of pain rather than instruments of pleasure. These are only a few of the many feelings that surface following hysterectomy and related surgeries. Uncovering and identifying the difficulties and emotions is certainly an important part of working out a solution. However, equally important is the level of commitment both you and your partner make toward achieving mutually satisfying sexual relations.

You really do reap what you sow. So keep that in mind when deciding how much effort you both are willing to put into this aspect of your relationship.

This chapter offers you a glimpse into the complexities of human sexual functioning and dysfunction. The information should serve as a more than adequate starting point toward attaining fulfilling sex.

Exercise, Nutrition and Healing

The last thing that you probably want to think about so soon after surgery is exercise. However, proper exercises done in moderation and with your physician's consent may help in your overall recovery.

Barring any serious complications, you will begin your exercise program the day after surgery. Your first exercise will be to get out of bed and go to the bathroom. Don't worry, you will not have to do this alone. The first time, a nurse will teach you how to move in and out of bed with minimum discomfort by using parts of the bed and stronger parts of your body to brace yourself. Once you've gotten in and out of bed a few times you'll feel more confident about taking on additional activities. Your next exercise should be to walk. As discussed in chapter 3, walking helps to get your bowels functioning, stave off boredom (to some extent) and get your muscles exercised and working. Begin taking short walks at first. If necessary, ask a nurse, family member or friend to assist you. When you feel comfortable with taking on more, then extend the distance.

Exercising in the hospital is somewhat easier than exercising at home, in part because you have medical people reminding you to do it and also because everything is conveniently located on your floor (meals are brought to you, the bathroom and shower are nearby and help is just a buzz away). Most homes are not set up in such a way as to make all your activities easily achievable (for example, bathrooms are often on a different level from the kitchen), and there are all sorts of people encouraging you to take it easy. Don't take these types of suggestions too seriously, try hard not to pamper yourself too much, in short get up and move!

The best approach to continuing your exercise program should be to confine yourself to one level (either upstairs or downstairs) for two weeks postoperatively. It is best to avoid stairs because climbing tends to stretch the incision area. In an ideal world, you would have someone there to help fetch and carry things. But if you are alone for a large part of the day take heed of the following suggestions:

> If you must use the stairs, make certain that you take care of everything you may want or need on that level before considering taking the stairs again.
>
> When you change levels, rest on that level for at least twenty to forty minutes.
>
> Prepare a sandwich, salad, or quick meal and a snack while in the kitchen. Then, when you are ready to return to the upper level, take the snack and something to drink up with you.
>
> For the first few days at home, try not to be alone when taking a shower. It is often more taxing than anticipated—it is helpful to have someone around to lend support if necessary.

After the third week following surgery you will probably begin to want to do more. You will be permitted to climb stairs now, so you will have more mobility. You might start out with some simple, gentle stretching exercises lasting a maximum of fifteen minutes and follow up with some walking. Do not exercise to the point of exhaustion (you don't get extra points or heal faster by being foolish).

To help you track your progress and/or problems it is wise to keep a chart. See table 7.

TABLE 7

Day	Activity	Duration	Comment
Monday	stretching	5 minutes	no problems
Tuesday	rest		
Wednesday	stretch/walk	10/15 minutes	no problems
Thursday	rest		
Friday	stretch/walk	15/15 minutes	challenging
Saturday	rest		
Sunday	stretch/walk	10/15 minutes	better

By keeping a chart of your activities, you can determine your progress as well as any problems that you may be having with specific activities. And as you feel yourself getting stronger, add suitable activities to round out your exercise program. If some activity seems to put unnecessary stress or pain on your body, stop it immediately, rest and see if the pain goes away. If the pain remains seek the counsel of a physician.

Exercise will not only help you to feel better emotionally, but it will also help you lessen your chances of developing osteoporosis. The point is, you must do some type of exercise so that your muscles do not atrophy and thereby weaken your overall body strength.

In order to get the most out of your exercise program, it is important not to overtax your joints and muscles. One way to prevent injury and to release overall body tension is professional massage. Often women's health clubs and YWCAs employ professionally trained masseuses. Finding someone good to give you a massage isn't difficult at all.

If you were in pain prior to surgery, you probably were not involved in a regular exercise program. Therefore, your muscles will probably need the support and relief achievable through massage. Therapeutic massage is the systematic manipulation of ligaments, muscles and connective tissue. A few benefits of massage are: reduction of overall body tension, increase of the blood flow to cells, an increase in flexibility and improved muscle tone. Physical and mental stress may inhibit the muscles from relaxing even when they are not in use. Constant muscle tension can seriously affect how you feel and how you perform. Consider massage as part of your rehabilitative exercise program and you'll get the maximum benefits from your efforts.

NUTRITION
Nutrition is also an important factor in promoting the healing process and maintaining good health. Many people assume that the food they eat provides them with the appropriate amounts of vitamins and minerals. The reality is that most people's daily diets do not contain the proper balance of protein, carbohydrates and fats. Most people get into trouble because of an excess in one of those particular groups, consuming too much sugar, caffeine, salt and alcohol. This, coupled with a

sedentary lifestyle because of the pain and discomfort associated with the disease, can spell disaster for a body low on reserves and in need of healing.

So how do you know what foods are good for you and which foods should be taken in moderation? Ask your physician and/or the hospital dietician to help you set up a meal plan that is appropriate for you. More frequently today hospitals provide this service to patients as a part of discharge procedure. In addition to the meal plan, use your own good common sense with regard to the amount of your intake of alcohol, caffeine, salt and sugar. The problems that these substances can cause have been pointed out in previous chapters and, while their elimination from your diet would be ideal, restricted use of these substances should be a minimum first step for you to take. Numerous books and papers are available to help you understand the value of nutrition. In addition, most cities have a growing number of nutritionists, so a one-time consultation with such a professional is a convenient and worthwhile approach. For women who live in rural areas, check with the hospital dietician prior to discharge for a list of qualified nutritionists.

An important point to remember is that the responsibility for your health is primarily up to you. You will have to take an interest and advocate for your best interests. In addition, most of the physicians, nurses, social workers, physical therapists and nutritionists at your disposal are extremely competent.

Voices of Experience

The following series of vignettes were developed as a result of interviews conducted with women who had a hysterectomy and in some cases an oophorectomy, men whose partners had this surgery and professionals who offer emotional support and professional help. While the details vary, many of the emotions expressed are shared. There are very specific illnesses for which hysterectomy may be performed. As you read these stories it will become clear that hysterectomy was not the appropriate treatment for all these women. Names have been changed and other identifying characteristics altered to protect their privacy.

ALEXIS
When Alexis was twenty-five she was told that she needed a hysterectomy. She had just completed law school and was scheduled to begin clerking at a prestigious New York city law firm. Her doctor told her that he had done all that he could to preserve her reproductive organs and that if she really wanted relief from the excruciating pain caused by her severe case of endometriosis, she should consent to having a hysterectomy and oophorectomy. He went on to say that performing the hysterectomy and oophorectomy was the only treatment that would guarantee her relief from debilitating pain. As the details of her story began to unfold it became clear that although surgery had taken place six years ago it continued to be a painful subject. She is a strong, intelligent woman with a sensitive demeanor. Her strength came about,

in part, out of her desire to survive the ordeal of this type of surgery at such an early age.

She calmly talks about her frustration with the inability of her doctor to control, if not cure, her endometriosis. She recounted her days in law school—how she had to use painkillers to sit through lectures and exams. Because she could tolerate the pain, she was able to complete law school and pass the bar exam. Alexis feels that she was cheated somehow. She adhered to the treatments that her doctor prescribed. She took Danazol, that wonderful drug which caused her skin to break out, gave her hot flushes, contributed fifteen pounds to her trim figure and added unsightly hair to her upper lip; she underwent successful laser surgery to remove all of the visible endometriomas, but most of all she gritted her teeth through the pain for thirty-six months only to be told that hysterectomy was her only option. So at twenty-five, with the world at her feet, engaged to a man she adored, she had to choose between years of intractable pain and permanent sterility.

Alexis decided to have the hysterectomy and oophorectomy because it seemed to be the one sure way to eliminate the pain she was experiencing. She didn't think it necessary to get a second opinion because she had known her physician since she was as child and trusted his judgment. She did, however, discuss her options with close friends and family and seemed to have their support.

The day of surgery Alexis was calm, but inquisitive. She asked the nurses for something to read that would describe what was going to happen to her during surgery and afterward. The brochure they offered was not adequate, so the attending resident offered a detailed explanation outlining the specifics of the surgery and discussed what she could expect following the procedure. The information was sufficient to sate her curiosity for that moment.

Alexis woke to an empty room, feeling quite a bit of pain. She asked the nurse to send in Jeff, her fiance, but was told that he had left the hospital immediately following surgery. It wasn't until later that Alexis began to realize that her once secure relationship was thrust onto rocky ground. For three days following surgery she received no communication from Jeff. He did not return her calls, he didn't visit and he didn't even send flowers. On the fourth day Jeff explained why he had stayed away. He felt robbed of the joy that comes with being a father, and he needed time to sort out whether his love for her was strong enough to handle this disappointment.

Clearly, this was the last thing that Alexis wanted or needed to hear. She couldn't believe the unfairness of the situation. With all she had been through, how could she be expected to deal with yet another crisis? To further complicate matters, she had incredible nightly sweating attacks and got very little sleep. She was depressed and weepy all of the time and generally wanted to crawl under the covers never to be seen again. A nurse came to her and explained that the hormonal changes that her body was going through were the cause of the night sweats, weepiness and mood swings. The nurse told her that estrogen would take care of these symptoms and that she should begin taking it immediately.

Alexis was discharged from the hospital after a ten-day stay. She was given a prescription for estrogen and Valium, instructions to take it easy and to return to her physician in six weeks time. In looking back, she thinks the surgery and subsequent hospital stay were the easiest part of the experience. The six months following the hysterectomy were months filled with anger, fear, depression and confusion.

Twelve weeks after surgery Alexis returned to work at the law firm. While at work she could feel whole, useful and competent. Although work distracted her from her situation, she had a terrible time coping with the hot flashes until her doctor upped the dosage of estrogen to 3.0 mg, the maximum amount. The Valium allowed her to get to sleep at night, but she had to take an increasingly higher dosage. Four months following surgery she had more problems than she ever bargained for: a turbulent and unfulfilling sex life, a failing relationship, chronic depression and a dependency on Valium.

Realizing that her life was in jeopardy, she took a six months leave of absence from her job, moved back home with her parents, found professional help for her dependency on Valium and sought out the help of a talented endocrinologist to help reduce the number and intensity of the hot flashes.

It took her five months to get herself together physically and psychologically. After extensive therapy she was able to come to terms with her hysterectomy and to withdraw gradually from the Valium. She was even better able to handle the hot flashes and flushes. Her body finally seemed to adjust to the sudden withdrawal of estrogen, and the flash/flush episodes had decreased dramatically. Finally, she could begin to focus on living her life again. But, even now, she has never been able to address the sexual problems resultant from the oophorectomy. In discussing this aspect of her life she is candid, but ashamed of her inability to function normally.

After her surgery she never felt aroused. Her desire for sex was nonexistent. She felt nothing physically or emotionally whenever she had sex with Jeff. She began to cry softly as she continued to describe the frustration she felt and continues to feel. Alexis, once a sexual, sensual woman, has been unable to reconnect herself sexually and feels unfeminine and unfulfilled. When asked if she ever considered consulting a sex therapist she retreats into silence and ends the interview.

Alexis' story is sad, not so much because of her choice to have a hysterectomy and oophorectomy, but because she has been unsuccessful in putting the sexual aspects of her life back on track. Sex for Alexis would probably not be as it was before surgery. However, with the proper help (sex therapist) and an understanding mate, her sexual experience might become more satisfying and fulfilling.

LISA

Lisa had been experiencing abdominal pain for at least twelve years. While it was annoying and uncomfortable, she was reticent to seek out help from her gynecologist until her symptoms reached a crisis level. She started having severe cramps several hours prior to her premier performance. Lisa is a talented dancer and choreographer of jazz works. She has great experience in biting the bullet in terms of dealing with and working through pain. She thought little about her pain, took some aspirin and began her warm-up exercises. She was determined to dance the opening performance, but at the last minute was unable even to crawl on stage. Once in the emergency room, the attending physician expressed alarm at the size of the growth in her uterus. Having had her tubes tied at thirty-two, she was certain that she wasn't pregnant. She was terrified of what might be growing inside her. After the sonogram and other tests, the physician asked her permission to perform an exploratory laparotomy with the possibility of a complete hysterectomy. Lisa agreed with one stipulation: that her own gynecologist be present and perform the surgery.

When Lisa woke up she felt strange. She found it difficult to focus on anything. She felt a bit sore and very drowsy. As she looked around the sterile hospital room she spotted her gynecologist. Dr. Arno took Lisa's hand in hers and said, "The good news is that the mass was not malignant, the bad news is that I was unable to save your uterus and one ovary." The mass was a benign fibroid tumor that had grown to be the size of a six-month fetus. In addition, an ovarian cyst on her right ovary had ruptured. Lisa felt relieved and happy. Part of the reason that she had neglected to contact her gynecologist during the last six months of pain and discomfort was her fear of cancer and death.

At forty she had no desire to have children. It was amazing to her how the removal of a relatively small organ could have such a positive impact on life.

Performing and creating were as important to Lisa as eating and breathing. Dr. Arno had given her back her life's blood. Lisa was no longer worn down by the many hours of daily pain, she no longer dreaded contemplating the next day's activities. She felt as if an incredible weight had been lifted. She was free and compelled to live her life with a vigor that was reminiscent of her twenties.

In addition to an improved dancing career, her sexual relationships were better than ever before. For the first time ever she was comfortable about her body and her sexuality. She felt no pain, no apprehension, no more guilt about having had her tubes tied. For years she had felt guilty about deciding not to have children. After all, she was brought up believing that strong, healthy and loving women were supposed to have children. It somehow seemed wrong that she should choose otherwise. Finally, the hysterectomy released her from any guilt that she had been feeling. This freedom allowed her to lose herself completely in her sexuality for the duration of intercourse. Lisa had spent most of her adult life committed to preventing conception and now finally she was pain free and had medical permission, if you will, *not* to conceive.

As she explained her feelings about the status of her reproductive capacity with tears in her eyes, she said, "Now I can really be me."

When asked what type and quality of information she received when she was in the hospital, she said flatly, "What information? There wasn't enough and what there was came too late." Lisa feels that by avoiding her abdominal pain for six months she relinquished her right to more complete information about her condition and any treatment that may have prevented the hysterectomy. However, on balance, in spite of her negligence, she thinks things worked out for the best.

CHELSEA

Chelsea was twenty-two years old when she began bleeding abnormally. She had always been a good student and a gregarious person. Because she was obese, she felt it necessary to make up for what she lacked in good appearance in academic achievement.

She remembered well the circumstances leading up to her decision to have a hysterectomy. During summer vacation, while she was visiting her aunt on Saginaw Island, she knew for certain that something was dreadfully wrong. She had been having quite a bit of abdominal pain and irregular bleeding for a few months, but had discounted it as being stress related. During the summer these symptoms escalated; the bleeding was extremely heavy. She had gastrointestinal problems as well. After some encouragement from her aunt, she made an appointment with her aunt's gynecologist.

As Chelsea began to describe her visit to the gynecologist's office, she started to wring her hands and look distressed. She said that it was the first time she realized that something was seriously wrong with her body. The doctor told her that the left ovary was very enlarged and the right ovary, while smaller, also felt abnormal, and suggested that she have surgery immediately to determine whether or not the ovaries were diseased. He went on to explain that he might have to remove her uterus and one or both of her ovaries if he found any malignancy. After what seemd to be a whirlwind consultation, Chelsea found herself in the hospital, recuperating from a hysterectomy and oophorectomy and scheduled for chemotherapy seventy-two hours following her initial consultation with the gynecologist.

It was difficult for Chelsea to come to terms with the harsh hand dealt to her. Granted she had the intelligence to take her to the highest heights, but she now felt that she had no chance to make a life for herself that resembled normalcy.

Because both ovaries were malignant and classified as "stage 4" (stage 4 means that both ovaries are affected and that there is some evidence of spread to other organs), chemotherapy was scheduled immediately. Chelsea had little or no time to consider the effects the surgery had on her body. She was more concerned with whether or not she would be able to survive this twist of fate.

Chelsea did not go back to school in September. Instead she battled with nausea, vomiting, hair loss, weight loss and depression caused by the chemotherapy treatments. As she spoke about this time in her life she exhibited a tremendous amount of pride—pride in having risen above the shock, heartache, pain and devastation of cancer and chemotherapy. And pleasure that she survived this physical and emotional trauma with a fair degree of success.

When asked about the effect the hysterectomy had on her life, she responded robustly, "It saved my life. We'd not be having this conversation if I hadn't had my uterus and ovaries removed. Although I wish that I had had more time to think about it and consider it, I am pleased that my gynecologist had the foresight and skill to act quickly. Having stage 4 ovarian cancer makes for interesting living. I am certain that my life expectancy is shorter than most women my age, but I am willing to live each breath of it to its fullest potential."

At the time of this interview, Chelsea had recently completed her residency in ophthalmology and was about to join an established practice in the Richmond, Virginia, area.

JENNIFER

Jennifer, an elegant, beautiful, gentle woman in her mid-forties is quiet, yet self-assured in her competence as a fashion designer. This is quite an accomplishment considering that several years ago she was a very different woman. It was about that time that her marriage began to fall apart, her ovarian cyst grew and accompanying it came more pain. And as if that weren't enough, she was waging a major battle against depression.

Jennifer had her hysterectomy because of a recurring problem with an ovarian cyst and a problem with urinary incontinence. There was no question in her mind as to whether this was the appropriate action to take. She trusted and hoped that this surgery would put an end to the nightmare that she was experiencing physically and emotionally.

The hysterectomy actually served as a turning point in her life. It occurred as she ended her marriage. She thought she was solving her health problems, but there was no neat and happy ending following surgery. Her urinary incontinence worsened and her physician seemed unable or unwilling to do anything else. After several more years of incontinence, Jenny found a urologist who was able to correct the urinary tract damage to the point in which she functioned normally. Step by step Jenny put her life back on track. She got professional help in dealing with her depression, and began building a life with a wonderful sensitive man who appreciated her. Once again, she could function as a responsible human being.

When asked if there was an area that was difficult in her life, she responded that "Sex is no longer a big part of my life." Prior to the gynecological problems she was able to enjoy sex with her husband. Now, however, she has problems with getting aroused, with lubrication and with orgasm. Sex is not the focal point in her relationship with her second husband. Although their sex life is not what she wants it to be, their high level of love manifested through other methods of intimacy helps her to put sex in perspective.

In this case, hysterectomy was not necessary. Hysterectomies should not ever be performed because of urinary incontinence and/or ovarian cysts. Ovarian cysts occur in women of all ages with a fair degree of regularity. Their mere presence is not a valid reason for the removal of the uterus (in this case a healthy organ) and both ovaries. What Jenny really needed was a therapist and a urologist, both of which she found after the hysterectomy. It is important to know which diseases are appropriate reasons for hysterectomy and which are not. Jenny was so frustrated by her dilemma and anxious for some resolution that she settled for unnecessary surgery.

JANE

Jane had a hysterectomy six months ago because of a severe case of endometriosis. Before surgery she had received several negative job performance reviews because she could not work five days out of each month. The pain she felt during those five days was overwhelming and debilitating. Darvocet, a prescription pain medication, became her constant companion, the only drug that could relieve the pain. Jane had had five separate surgeries to remove various endometriosis implants. But because her case was so severe—the previous surgeries had not eliminated the problem or even made the disease more manageable— her physician advised the removal of both her ovaries and her uterus. He pointed out that the hysterectomy would not solve the problem, but rather make it more manageable and less painful.

Jane accepted her physician's suggestion as her decision primarily because she was in too much pain and discomfort to take the time to seek a second opinion. She anticipated that the pain would cease, the disease process would end and her life would once again be normal. Following surgery, new problems began to surface one by one. Hot flushes, night sweats and depression occurred at the same time, more overwhelming because she had not been given information prior to surgery regarding the possibility and likelihood of these symptoms. Fortunately, her physician was quick to call in an endocrinologist to help address the estrogen withdrawal problems. Through the use of Bellergal (a sympathetic nervous system inhibitor) and Provera (a natural progestin), Jane's problems were under control within a month's time.

Once the hormonal problems cleared up she could proceed with her life full speed. Physically, she was able to work out daily and take part in activities that previously had been too taxing and painful. Sexually, she felt great because she could finally relax enough to enjoy intercourse. Prior to the surgery she had experienced so much pain that she couldn't relax during lovemaking. Because all of the other aspects of her life were once again in balance, she was on top of the world emotionally. In Jane's case, even though the hysterectomy and oophorectomy did not guarantee that the endometriosis was cured, the surgery succeeded in making the disease more manageable and therefore improved the quality of her life.

BETH

Six years ago, when Beth was thirty-three years old, she had a hysterectomy for cervical cancer. She remembers the events leading up to the surgery quite vividly. It was time for her annual checkup, and as part of that checkup a Pap smear was taken. Beth never expected to hear anything from her gynecologist because in the past the results had always been normal. However, she remembers the intensity of the voice on the other end of the phone and urgency in it. Her doctor pulled no punches. She came out with the news . . . "Your Pap smear was classified 5 which means that you have invasive cervical cancer. It is important for us to operate immediately to determine how extensive the cancer is." It felt as if a ton of bricks had fallen on her head and then someone had punched her in the stomach. She was disoriented, yet coherent enough to know the import of the situation.

Surgery was scheduled. Somehow the entire process lacked the drama and urgency of a Ben Casey or Marcus Welby rerun. Beth expected the world to stop and sigh or acknowledge that a horrible fate had been dealt to her, but there was none of that. Surgery came and went without so much as a small roar. Following surgery, her gynecologist explained that it had been necessary to remove her uterus because the cancer had spread, but that her ovaries were still intact. All the cancer had been cleaned out and there was little chance of recurrence.

Beth speaks about her hysterectomy as if it were some sort of religious experience. She sees the hysterectomy as a turning point in her life. For Beth, the hysterectomy gave her a second chance. She looked at her life, assessed its flaws and its good points and made changes to improve its quality.

Beth had few problems following surgery. Her recuperation period was minimal, her emotional spirits high and she felt as if she had conquered the world. I asked her during the interview to take a closer look at her life following the surgery and her reply was, "Of course, there were problems, but I refused to dwell on those things that made me unhappy." She spoke about consulting with a therapist after the operation to help with some adjustment problems relating to the cancer. Those sessions lasted eight weeks and addressed her problems successfully.

Her advice to others who may be undergoing a hysterectomy is simple and straightforward . . . "Keep a positive attitude, make sure you've got a good surgeon and have a good support system in place."

ANNIE

Annie is fifty-five and had a hysterectomy two months prior to our interview. A spry woman, she has very little in her life to be happy about. She had the hysterectomy because she was tired of the sporadic nature of her periods. She was unwilling to wait for a few years until the menopause process ended. She says that she faked being in pain as well as other symptoms in order to have her doctor perform the hysterectomy. She tells her story with great pride—pride that she, a simple woman, was able to fool such a learned man. Annie was sure that the hysterectomy would take care of her sadness and depression, but it did not. She is still very unhappy, even more so since the surgery. Annie equates this operation with having had her child thirty-five years ago. Just as she thought that a child would give her joy and improve her marriage back then, she thought a hysterectomy would work its magic. But each time it did not turn out as she wanted.

When asked if there were specific problems associated with the surgery, she responded that it was difficult to sort out what started when. Sex had never been an important part of their marriage. Her husband had taken numerous lovers over the years to satisfy his desires. She had never worked or been responsible for herself and her biggest fear was that she would have to become responsible for her life. Annie thinks that she has been faking living her life since the early days of her marriage. She feels that she has run out of time and excuses. However, when asked about the possibility of therapy, she became enraged at the suggestion that there is anything wrong with her behavior. She seemed to take great pleasure in the misfortunes of her life and gets some enjoyment from talking about her unhappiness.

MEN SPEAK ABOUT HYSTERECTOMY

RICHARD

Richard was the last person to know about his wife's hysterectomy. Janet, his wife, a woman in her late fifties, was worried that he would lose interest in her and seek out other women. It wasn't until a few days before surgery that he found out about the hysterectomy and the possibility of ovarian cancer.

When the doctor discussed the pathologist's findings with Richard and Janet, they both knew that time was sparse and hope was nil. Janet had stage 4 ovarian cancer with wide area spread. At that point, the aftermath of hysterectomy was not the issue. Saving Janet's life was uppermost in everyone's mind.

When Richard talked about that time in his life he seemed sad. He said that there was never a time when he felt so helpless. The chemotherapy treatments following the operation made Janet constantly uncomfortable. She was totally depressed when all of her hair fell out and it was about that time she began to withdraw from him altogether (emotionally and sexually). It was then that Richard decided to pull out all the stops.

He didn't want Janet to be alone, nor was he ready to lose her companionship. He waged an all-out war to help convince Janet that she was still the woman he adored and loved, that his life was richer with her in it (even though the medical problems made life more complicated), and that she had a responsibility to love him as long as she was able. Because Janet did not feel comfortable having intercourse, Richard decided that cuddling, massaging and gentle caressing were ways to help make her feel feminine and desirable. It was also a way for him to feel useful. After a few months of chemotherapy and radiation, it became clear to everyone that Janet was going to die. When asked if he changed any of his habits after hearing the news of impending death, he said, "I have always loved Janet, but I have not always shown it. I wish that I could take away all her doubts about my feelings for her. I will continue to be with her until her last breath, and I will make her death peaceful and less lonely. After all, isn't that what unconditional love is about?"

(Janet died two days after this interview.)

JIM

Jim, twenty-eight, had been living with Donna for three years. He thought that their relationship was a good one. But now that Donna could not have his children, he wasn't too sure how he felt about her. Jim was embarrassed by his feelings but at least he was being honest. His hopes and dreams for a family were shattered by this awful surgery and he didn't like it one bit.

He began drinking heavily after Donna came home from the hospital. He avoided being near her, and found activities outside of his home to occupy his time. He knew that his actions hurt Donna, but he wouldn't or couldn't do anything to change them. He didn't want to touch her sexually because the thought of it made him uncomfortable. To Jim, she was different, not the woman he had fallen in love with.

This estrangement went on for over a year. Jim's behavior became more and more abusive. Finally, Donna asked him to leave and he did. He soon found that life without her was not good either. So he started seeing a counselor to help him understand his feelings and behavior.

Over the next year, he was able to identify his problems where Donna was concerned. He learned that his feelings had very little to do with her inability to have children, but rather his inability to identify her as a female because she now lacked reproductive organs. To him, making love to her would be no different than making love to a man, and the idea repulsed him. With the help of his therapist, Jim was able to work on his difficulties with gender identification. However, by the time Jim got to a point where he could communicate with Donna, it was too late. Donna had recovered from surgery and Jim's abusive treatment and was stronger than ever. While she was willing to talk to Jim, she was not willing to consider a reconciliation.

Jim is sad that he handled the situation so badly. But he feels stronger and more sure of who he is personally and sexually. He is certain that his next relationship will last because of his new strength.

ERNESTO

Ernesto, forty-one, had been married to Luisa for seven years. Theirs was a happy, solid marriage. They were proud of their six-year-old daughter and enjoyed a rewarding and comfortable lifestyle.

When asked how he felt about Luisa's hysterectomy, Ernesto said, "I was hopeful that the hysterectomy would succeed in sparing her from the pain she had been suffering for so long (about one year). I felt it was a chance to do something definitive, concrete about her discomfort.

"My only apprehensions about the hysterectomy were for Luisa's happiness. That was the only thing that I cared about. During her past medical problems, we had gone without sex for many months so I knew it was possible to have a happy marriage with a sporadic sex life."

He and Luisa went through some rocky periods. When she felt weak (emotionally and/or physically) she would think about throwing in the towel. But Ernesto knew that she needed her privacy, a time to "lick her wounds" and brood, so he gave her the necessary space. Luisa usually initiated those times of isolation. As long as Ernesto and Luisa were together, he could try to pull her out of isolation. He used those opportunities to involve her in projects in and outside of the home.

Prior to the hysterectomy, Luisa had had a series of surgeries that put her out of sexual commission for months at a time. A novel aspect of lovemaking was that Luisa's hot flashes/flushes would come on so intensely that even when they both were sexually aroused Luisa would become distracted and unable to proceed. Imbalance in sexual advances was another problem for Ernesto. In "normal" times, "I would know whether my advances were welcomed or not because Luisa would respond. After the hysterectomy and oophorectomy it would take fifteen to thirty minutes of foreplay to get Luisa to the point where she herself could tell whether or not she was interested in sex. This was terribly confusing to me."

Sex has improved for them because the hot flashes have declined from every ten minutes or so to a few times a week. The disruption they caused has been nearly eliminated. "Luisa has also become more secure in her self-image as a sexual being. She doesn't feel quite so fraudulent now." (Luisa makes love because she wants to and not out of duty.) The fear of pain receded, and reduced her apprehension around having sex. "I got used to the idea of taking the initiative for a longer period of time before getting confirmation from Luisa that she was in the mood too."

The hysterectomy has had very little negative impact on their relationship. Ernesto said proudly, "Our relationship has always been rock solid. The raging hormonal battles in Luisa's body after the hysterectomy meant that she had larger mood swings than usual. I had to bite my tongue and try to moderate the mood swings rather than react to them. I couldn't respond to her anger with a fit of my own. She had a lot of things to be angry about and sometimes I was the only target available. But I knew that she really loved me and always did love me and that her anger would pass once she vented some of her justifiable frustration."

Ernesto offers this advice to others in this situation. "Look beyond the surface reason for the arguments and/or difficulties. Often it is simply a lightning rod for the anger the woman feels over the raw deal she's been dealt. Also, men should have hope, because things in fact do gradually improve. Situations that would be intolerable if they showed no signs of ending, do in fact become easier and more normal."

THOSE WHO HELP

The following two women help women and couples deal with the effects of hysterectomy and/or oophorectomy.

Catherine, a young woman in her thirties, had a hysterectomy and oophorectomy two years ago. She was lucky enough to live in an area where pre- and posthysterectomy workshops were available. She found the workshops invaluable to her overall recovery, but the cost was prohibitive. She decided to put together a self-help group for women who were going through this type of surgery. She wanted to offer support, information and referrals to women at no charge.

Catherine believes that women have to learn to supplement the information available from their physicians. "Sometimes doctors don't have the time to give you all the information available to help make your posthysterectomy life manageable. Sometimes they just don't have the information we need because it falls into a different medical specialty. Whatever the reason, if we as health consumers can help each other through support groups and referral bases, then we've accomplished a great deal."

Some of the more common problems Catherine hears about are: loss of sexual urge, vaginal dryness and sensitivity, depression and hot flashes. "It has been very helpful for women to come together and discuss common problems, swap possible solutions and be listened to with a sympathetic ear."

Catherine is adamant about facilitating a positive group. She is not opposed to gripe sessions, but always points out the necessity for finding a path toward resolution. "I'm not a trained therapist, but I've learned a lot through my experiences. I don't have to be a therapist to offer hope."

Dr. Lucy Waletzky, a psychiatrist and codirector of the Medical Illness Counseling Center agreed to be interviewed on the impact of hysterectomy on women and their partners. A significant part of Dr. Waletzky's time is spent helping women with sexual dysfunction problems.

When asked what impact hysterectomy had on relationships, Dr. Waletzky said, "There are a certain number of couples who have a more difficult time following hysterectomy, there are a certain percentage that experience no change in the quality of their relationship, and there are a percentage of couples in which the relationship improves." Dr. Waletzky believes that the effect on a relationship depends on the state of the relationship and sexual activity prior to the surgery as well as the reason for the hysterectomy and/or oophorectomy. (If for example, a woman in her fifties who has had a number of children is told that hysterectomy is the best option for her abnormal bleeding and pain; she will be free of pain following surgery and can resume her normal activities. However, if a twenty-year-old unmarried woman has uterine cancer, her emotional response to the surgery may be extreme.)

Another factor that affects relationships is how the man perceives the woman following hysterectomy. Some men see women as being de-sexed. It is crucial for men not to pretend that everything is all right. They should seek out counseling to try to work through their problems with gender identification.

Other factors that affect relationships are the general psychological health of the couple, and the stability of their relationship. In strong relationships, the couple weathers the storm and often becomes even stronger. But in weaker relationships, the problems and stresses that come with hysterectomy may be too much.

Hysterectomy has brought some couples closer together. Often when the fear of pregnancy is removed, couples can relax and enjoy more sexual freedom.

When asked what advice she would give to couples, Dr. Waletzky said, "It is never too late to correct sexual dysfunction problems. I have been able to help very young women as well as women into their seventies. There is always hope."

PHYSICIANS

A dozen physicians in the Washington, D.C., metropolitan area were asked how they handled their patients who were facing hysterectomy and possible oophorectomy. The physicians who seemed to be the most willing to answer questions like those listed in chapter 1 were the specialists in infertility, oncology and/or those physicians connected with a teaching hospital. Most of them stated that they were pleased to have informed patients who were willing to take some responsibility for their own health care. They added, though, that the problem with well informed patients is that often they don't know as much as they think they do, and don't understand *all* the nuances of a particular procedure. All of these doctors were adamant that communication was almost as important a skill as their medical knowledge. They stressed the importance of answering questions, addressing fears and being accessible when possible. They also stressed the importance of women not abusing this accessibility. Sometimes when a woman is in the midst of a medical crisis, she will call her physician when the appropriate person to call might be a friend or counselor. And while sometimes it is possible to serve in this capacity, it is not the physician's primary role or responsibility. Physicians who specialize in infertility have found that adding social workers to their medical team has been extremely useful in directing patients to the proper caregiver. And although most of the physicians questioned were willing to have patient participation, a few were not at all interested in such involvement. One said flatly, "I am the doctor. I know how to handle gynecological diseases and disorders and I have the degree. I do not want some patient telling me how to do my job."

He went on to explain that he would not treat someone who came into his office with a list of questions; he would send such a woman away. When I asked why he'd react so strongly, he said that people are litigious now. "If someone even thinks that you may have acted inappropriately then they litigate. I think that it is a warning signal of later problems if they come in asking questions." This same physician felt that patients were becoming "soft." In the old days "there was not all this hand holding and coddling stuff; nowadays everyone is overly sensitive and demands special care. All I want to do is practice good medicine . . . leave the coddling and hand holding to the psychiatrists."

Although the number of doctors interviewed is small, it represents the physician population at large.

This guide can help you cope with the medical maze of activity surrounding hysterectomy. Use it as a guide along with your own common sense. Only then can you be sure that you are handling this experience in a way that is best for you.

A P P E N D I X   1
G L O S S A R Y   O F   T E R M S

ADENOMYOSIS is a condition in which the endometrial tissue (lining of the uterus) penetrates the uterine wall making it thick, spongy and tender. Abdominal pain and prolonged, heavy periods are the most common symptoms.

ADHESIONS are formed when two or more organs or surfaces that are ordinarily separate become connected to each other by means of a thin fibrous band. While adhesions are most often caused by surgery, they can also occur following certain pelvic disorders.

ANALGESIC is any drug that relieves pain.

ANAPROX is an analgesic and anti-inflammatory drug that inhibits the synthesis of prostaglandins, which cause the contraction of the uterus and other smooth muscles. This drug is often prescribed to women who have mild to moderate pain.

ANTIPROSTAGLANDINS are a group of drugs that work to inhibit the synthesis of prostaglandins. In addition to causing smooth muscles to contract, prostaglandins are believed to have an effect on the female hormones sometimes causing an imbalance.

BELLERGAL is a drug that is often given to women experiencing menopausal symptoms. It is thought that hot flashes, night sweats, etc. occur partly as a result of the hyperactivity of the sympathetic and parasympathetic nervous systems. Bellergal, which is a sympathetic inhibitor, is often successful in relieving the symptoms.

BENIGN refers to the noncancerous status of a lump or mass that has been biopsied.

BIOFEEDBACK is a scientific technique that allows you to monitor your own body functions, such as heart rate, skin temperature, muscle tension, etc. and to use that information (feedback) to control and alter those functions.

BIOPSY involves the removal and scientific examination of tissue from a living body to determine its disease status.

CANCER is a term that encompasses a group of diseases in which there is a transformation of normal cells into malignant ones. The malignant cells continue to grow in an abnormal and destructive way.

CERVIX is the oval-shaped organ located at the uppermost end of the vaginal canal. It is the organ that separates the vagina from the uterus.

CHLAMYDIA is a bacterial infection which causes such symptoms as thick yellow vaginal discharge, itching and cervical irritation.

CLIMACTERIC refers to a change from a reproductive to a non-reproductive phase in women. Unless surgically induced, this phase usually occurs from thirty-five to sixty-five years of age.

CLONIDINE is a drug that is being used in research settings on women experiencing menopausal symptoms. Hot flashes, and night sweats, may occur partly as a result of hyperactivity of the sympathetic and parasympathetic nervous systems. Clonidine, which is a sympathetic inhibitor, has been somewhat effective in relieving the symptoms.

CONIZATION refers to the removal of a tissue sample from the cervix usually in the shape of a cone.

CONTRAINDICATION indicates a danger of a particular drug or treatment.

CORTICAL BONE TISSUE is the solid and dense bone material that surrounds the inner bone. When osteoporosis occurs, this protective bone becomes dangerously thin, making a woman more prone to fractures and breaks.

DANAZOL is a synthetic androgen (male hormone) that inhibits the output of hormones from the pituitary gland. When used in treating endometriosis, Danazol alters the normal and abnormal endometrial tissue so that it becomes inactive and shrinks.

DEPRESSION is an abnormal response to events (positive or negative) due to distorted thoughts about those events. It is a sadness or melancholy that is disproportionate to a particular set of events.

DIABETES is a disease of the pancreas, characterized by the production of excessive amounts of urine. The major risk factors for adult-onset diabetes are heredity and obesity.

DYSPARUNIA refers to painful intercourse.

ENDOCRINOLOGY is the study of the disorders of the glands of internal secretion (endocrine glands).

ENDOMETRIOSIS is a condition in which endometrial tissue (tissue from the lining of the uterus) begins to grow in various sites outside the uterus. These growths commonly attach themselves to the ovaries, fallopian tubes, bladder and rectum as well as other parts in the abdominal cavity. These growths function as if they continue to be a part of the uterine lining, thickening and bleeding into the pelvic cavity each month in accordance with the ovarian cycle.

ESTROGEN is a generic term for estrus-producing compounds, the female hormones. Estradiol, estriol and estrone are included in this definition.

ESTROGEN DEPENDENT is a term applied to a condition or disease in which the growth of the disease is directly linked to the presence of estrogen.

FALLOPIAN TUBES operate as a vehicle to transport the egg from the ovary to the uterus.

FIBROCYSTIC BREAST DISEASE is a term used to categorize most diseases of the breast that are not malignant. Women with fibrocystic disease have increased levels of estrogens during the second half of the menstrual cycle. It is thought that the fibrocystic disease is an abnormal response to the higher estrogen levels. The symptoms that are most frequently reported are painful swelling of the breast and the presence of cysts.

FIBROIDS refer to common uterine growths composed of connective and muscle fiber which originate from the wall of the uterus. Almost all diagnosed cases of fibroids (leiomyoma in medical terminology) are benign.

FOLLICLE STIMULATING HORMONE, also referred to as FSH, is a hormone produced by the pituitary gland to stimulate the maturation of egg cells in the ovary.

GONAD refers to an organ which produces sex cells (the ovary in a female and the testis in the male).

GONADOTROPIN is a hormone capable of promoting gonadal growth and function, such as the pituitary hormones FSH and LH.

GONOCOCCUS is a bacterial organism that usually attacks the mucous membranes of the genital and urinary organs, producing inflammation and pus. In adults the disease is contracted through sexual intercourse with an infected person. Gonorrhea is the more common term for this bacterial infection.

HEALTH JOURNAL is a tool used by patients to record and document their symptoms. This information, when discussed with the physician, gives a more complete history.

HORMONAL REPLACEMENT THERAPY involves the use of hormones (estrogens and progesterones) to control and prevent symptoms of estrogen deficiency such as: hot flashes, vaginal atrophy and osteoporosis.

HOT FLASH refers to the subjective feeling that a woman has prior to the physical measurable temperature change, the HOT FLUSH. The hot flash usually precedes the hot flush by approximately forty-five seconds.

HYSTERECTOMY involves the removal of the uterus either through the vagina or through the abdomen. A total hysterectomy refers to the removal of the uterus and the cervix. In a radical hysterectomy the uterus, the upper third of the vagina and the supporting ligaments are removed. In a subtotal hysterectomy the uterus is removed, but the cervix is left in place.

IMAGERY or creative visualization is a method of using your imagination to create a specific scenario in your life. Within the boundaries of your mind you set the scene using a stressful situation in your life, write the dialogue and determine the outcome. Research psychologists believe that the use of imagery may in fact release a hormone contained in the body that stimulates the immune system. In addition, the very use of imagery can be effective in reducing the levels of stress.

INFERTILITY is the inability of a woman to conceive and/or to carry a fetus to full term.

KEGEL EXERCISES were developed originally to help women who suffered from urinary stress incontinence, a condition in which small amounts of urine are released if a woman coughs, sneezes, jumps or has an orgasm. The exercises work on the pubococcygeal muscle (PC muscle), the muscle which cradles and supports the pelvic organs.

LAPAROSCOPY is a diagnostic tool used to examine the abdominal cavity. An incision is made in the navel and a slender instrument, a laparascope, is inserted to examine the pelvic cavity.

LAPAROTOMY is a term used for a procedure in which an incision is made in the abdominal wall in order to carry out certain types of major surgery. Such surgeries might include removal of fibroids, removal of endometriomas, hysterectomy and salpingo-oophorectomy.

LESION refers to any abnormal change in the structure of an organ or tissue.

LIBIDO refers to the sexual desire derived, in part, from the instinctive biological drives.

LUTENIZING HORMONE, also referred to as LH, is produced by the pituitary gland to stimulate the ovaries in the second half of the menstrual cycle.

MALIGNANT is a term used to describe the cancerous state of biopsied cells.

MAMMOGRAPHY is an X-ray technique used to examine breast tissue for irregularities.

MENOPAUSE occurs when the menstrual cycle stops, usually when a woman reaches mid-life. Surgical menopause refers to the cessation of the menstrual cycle as a result of the removal of the ovaries and the uterus.

MIGRAINE refers to a severe headache that is often, but not always, limited to one side of the head. Frequently this type of headache is accompanied by nausea and vomiting.

MOTRIN is an analgesic and anti-inflammatory drug that inhibits the synthesis of prostaglandins. This drug is often given to women with mild to moderate pain.

MYOMECTOMY is a surgical procedure in which all fibroids are removed without removing the uterus. This type of surgery is a preferred first course invasive treatment for fibroids.

NIGHT SWEATS are a variation on the flash/flush episode except that they occur during the night while a woman is sleeping. The bed linens are usually soaked in perspiration and the woman's sleep is usually disturbed for the remainder of the evening.

ONCOLOGY is the study of tumors.

OSTEOPOROSIS refers to the loss of bone mass or thinning of the bones. Osteoporosis has been linked directly to estrogen decline and withdrawal.

OVARIES are the oval-shaped organs located on opposite sides of the uterus. The ovaries have two basic functions; the production of estrogen and progesterone and the formation of ova.

PAP SMEAR is a simple screening test performed in the doctor's office. Cells are gently removed from the cervix and sent to the lab for evaluation. If the results are in the normal range, there is no need for concern. However, if the cells are abnormal, further tests are required to either rule out or verify malignancy.

PELVIC INFLAMMATORY DISEASE, also known as PID, is a pelvic infection that may involve the ovaries, fallopian tubes and pelvic connective tissue. Many women are rendered infertile as a result of this disease.

PERITONEUM is the membrane that lines the walls of the abdominal and pelvic cavity.

PITUITARY GLAND is one of the endocrine glands located at the base of the brain.

PONSTEL is an analgesic and anti-inflammatory drug that inhibits the synthesis of prostaglandins. This drug is given to women experiencing mild to moderate pain.

PROGESTOGEN is a synthetic hormone which acts like progesterone, the female hormone produced in the second half of the normal menstrual cycle.

PROSTAGLANDINS are a group of naturally occurring fatty acids that stimulate contraction of the uterus and other smooth muscles. Prostaglandins are also believed to affect the activity of certain female hormones.

PUBOCOCCYGEAL MUSCLE, also known as the PC muscle, is the muscle that cradles or supports the pelvic organs.

SALPINGO-OOPHORECTOMY involves the surgical removal of one (unilateral) or both (bilateral) ovaries and fallopian tubes.

SEXUAL DYSFUNCTION refers to problems that disrupt normal sexual functioning. These problems may be physical or psychological in nature, or a combination of the two. Sexual dysfunction is not a permanent disorder, but usually requires the assistance of a trained therapist to overcome.

THROMBOPHLEBITIS is the inflammation of a vein associated with blood clot formation.

TRABECULAR BONE is the tissue located inside the cortical bone. This tissue is more porous and gives the appearance of being more loosely structured and therefore more easily affected by bone loss.

URINARY STRESS INCONTINENCE is a condition in which small amounts of urine are released when a woman coughs, sneezes, jumps or has an orgasm. This condition can usually be remedied by strengthening the PC muscle using Kegel exercises.

UTERUS is the pear-shaped muscular organ in which the fertilized egg is embedded and the developing fetus is nourished. Between puberty and menopause, the uterine lining goes through a monthly cycle of growth and discharge known as the menstrual cycle.

VAGINAL ATROPHY is a condition in which the vaginal walls begin to thin, become more sensitive. This condition is often linked to a lack of sufficient estrogen in women who have experienced menopause (surgical or natural).

VAGINAL MYOGRAPH is a spoollike soft plastic device shaped like a dumb-bell which when inserted vaginally can provide both sex therapist and client with information about the PC muscle activity. The vaginal myograph is used in conjunction with the regular EMG (electro-myographic) biofeedback device.

A P P E N D I X   2
R E S O U R C E S

NEWSLETTERS

Broomstick, Options for Women over Forty
3543 18th Street
San Francisco, California 94110
This is a bi-monthly publication by, for and about women over forty, with a feminist orientation.

HERS (Hysterectomy Educational Resources)
422 Bryn Mawr Avenue
Bala Cynwyd, Pennsylvania 19004
(215) 667-7757
This organization publishes a quarterly newsletter and provides information about hysterectomy and oophorectomy.

Hot Flash: Newsletter for Midlife and Older Women
c/o Dr. Jane Porcino
School of Allied Health Professions
SUNY
Stony Brook, New York 11794
This is quarterly publication devoted to promoting wellness in the post-menopausal woman.

Medical Self Care
P.O. Box 717
Inverness, California 94937
This is a quarterly magazine directed to all aspects of health. There is a particular focus on promoting self-care.

Midlife Wellness
Center for Climacteric Studies
University of Florida
901 N. West 8th Avenue, Suite B1
Gainesville, Florida 32601

This is a quarterly journal dealing with all aspects of menopause and mid-life wellness. Although the journal is geared toward the health care professional, the material is presented in a manner easily understood by the lay person.

Nutrition Action
Center for Science in the Public Interest
1755 S Street N.W.
Washington, D.C. 20009

This is a monthly publication which provides practical nutritional information to the lay consumer.

Planetree Health Resource Center
2040 Webster Street
San Francisco, California 94115
(415) 346-4636

This center will conduct medical searches using Medline and other professional data bases for a small fee. They also have bibliographies on many health topics, and they sell health related books.

PMZ (Post Menopausal Zest) Newsletter
c/o Volcano Press
330 Ellis Street, Dept. MN
San Francisco, California 94102

This publication is an annual update by Dr. Sadja Greenwood on the most current medical information regarding menopause, hormonal therapy and general post-menopausal health.

ORGANIZATIONS

American Association of Sex Educators, Counselors and Therapists (AASECT)
11 Dupont Circle N.W.
Washington, D.C. 20036
(202) 462-1171

This Association can help put you in contact with qualified sex therapists in your area.

American Board of Clinical Biofeedback
2424 Dempster Street
Des Plaines, Illinois 60016
(312) 827-0440

For additional information on the vaginal myograph—(800) 537-3779

Boston Women's Health Book Collective
465 Mt. Auburn Street
Watertown, Massachusetts 02172
This is a non-profit organization devoted to education about women and health.

Breast Cancer Advisory Service
Rose Kushner, Director
P.O. Box 224
Kensington, Maryland 20895

Cancer Information Service
National Cancer Hotline 1 (800) 4CA-NCER
This number is answered from 8:00 a.m. to midnight

Endometriosis Association
Mary Lou Ballweg, President
P.O. Box 92187
Milwaukee, Wisconsin 53202

National Library of Medicine
Medlars Management Section
8600 Rockville Pike
Bethesda, Maryland 20209
This organization is responsible for the on-line Medline service which is available through most large hospitals and medical schools. In addition, there are seven regional medical libraries listed below. These libraries will be able to conduct an on-line search for you for a fee.

REGIONAL LIBRARIES

Greater Northeastern Regional Medical Library Program
New York Academy of Medicine
2 East 103rd Street
New York, NY 10029
(212) 876-8763
States Served: CT, DE, MA, ME, NH, NJ, NY, PA, RI, VT, and Puerto Rico

Southeastern Atlantic Regional Medical Library Services
University of Maryland
Health Sciences Library
111 South Greene Street
Baltimore, MD 21201
(301) 528-2855; (800) 638-6093

States Served: AL, FL, GA, MD, MS, NC, SC, TN, VA, WV, and District of Columbia

Greater Midwest Regional Medical Library
University of Illinois at Chicago
Library of the Health Sciences
Health Sciences Center
Chicago, IL 60680
(312) 996-2464
States Served: IA, IL, IN, KY, MI, MN, ND, OH, SD, WI

Midcontinental Regional Medical Library Program
University of Nebraska
Medical Center Library
42nd & Dewey Avenue
Omaha, NE 68105
(402) 559-4326
States Served: CO, KS, MO, NE, UT, WY

South Central Regional Medical Library Program
University of Texas
Health Science Center at Dallas
5323 Harry Hines Boulevard
Dallas, TX 75235
(214) 688-2085
States Served: AR, LA, NM, OK, TX

Pacific Northwest Regional Health Sciences Library Service
Health Sciences Library
University of Washington
Seattle, WA 98195
(206) 543-8262
States Served: AK, ID, MT, OR, WA

Pacific Southwest Regional Medical Library Service
UCLA Biomedical Library
Center for the Health Sciences
Los Angeles, CA 90024
(213) 825-1200
States Served: AZ, CA, HI, NV

National Women's Health Network
224 Seventh Street SE
Washington, D.C. 20024
This is a national organization that serves as a clearinghouse for women's health

issues. The Network also publishes a newsletter regarding health and lobbying issues.

National Chronic Pain Outreach
8222 Wycliffe Court
Manassas, VA 22110

This is a national network of self-help groups offering emotional support and practical help to individuals and families trying to cope with any chronic pain situation.

Resolve, Inc.
National Headquarters
P.O. Box 474
Belmont, MA 02178

SIECUS (Sex Information and Education Council of the US)
84 Fifth Avenue
New York, NY 10011

SIECUS has many bibliographies on sex-related topics. Write to them for a complete listing and an order form.

B I B L I O G R A P H Y

HYSTERECTOMY AND MENOPAUSE

Cherry, Sheldon H. *The Menopause Myth*. New York: Ballantine, 1976.

Cutler, Winnifred Berg, Garcia, Celso-Ramon, and Edwards, David A. *Menopause: A Guide for Women and the Men Who Love Them*. New York: W. W. Norton & Company, 1983.

Donohugh, D. *The Middle Years, A Physical Guide to Your Body, Emotions and Life Challenges*. Sanders.

Fromer, Margot. *Menopause*. New York: Pinnacle Books, 1985.

Greenwood, Sadja. *Menopause, Naturally*. San Francisco: Volcano, 1984.

Guistine, L.G. and Keffer, L.J. *Understanding Hysterectomy*. New York: Walker, 1979.

Jameson, Deedee and Schwalb, Roberta. *Everywoman's Guide to Hysterectomy*. Englewood Cliffs, NJ: Prentice-Hall.

Lauersen, M.D., Niels and Whitney, Steven. *It's Your Body*. New York: Playboy Press Paperbacks, 1977.

London, Mel. *Second Spring*. Emmaus, PA: Rodale, 1982.

Morgan, Suzanne. *Coping with a Hysterectomy*. New York: Dial, 1982.

Notelovitz, M. & Ware, M. *Stand Tall! The Informed Woman's Guide for Preventing Osteoporosis*. Gainesville, FL: Triad, 1982.

Nugent, Nancy. *Hysterectomy*. Garden City, NY: Doubleday, 1976.

Page, Jane. *The Other Awkward Age*. Berkeley, CA: Ten Speed Press, 1977.

Reitz, Rosetta. *Menopause, A Positive Approach*. Radnor, PA: Chilton Books, 1977.

Rose, Louisa. *The Menopause Book*. New York: Hawthorne Books, 1977.

Seaman, Barbara and Seaman, Gideon. *Women and the Crisis in the Sex Hormones*. New York: Bantam, 1977.

Weideyer, Paula. *Menstruation and Menopause*. New York: Dell, 1975.

Wise Budoff, Penny. *No More Hot Flashes and Other Good News*. New York: Warner, 1983.

SEXUALITY

Barbach, L.G. *For Yourself—The Fulfillment of Female Sexuality*. New York: Doubleday, 1975.

Barbach, L.G. *For Each Other*. New York: Doubleday, 1984.

Belliveau, F., & Richter, I. *Understanding Human Sexual Inadequacy*. New York: Bantam, 1970.

Bonaparte, M. *Female Sexuality*. International Universities Press, 1953.

Boston's Women's Health Collective. *The New Our Bodies, Ourselves*. New York: Simon and Schuster, 1984.

Carrera, M. *Sex: The Facts, the Acts, and Your Feelings*. New York: Crown, 1981.

Comfort, A. *The Joy of Sex*. New York: Crown, 1972.

Downing, G. *The Massage Book*. New York: Random House, 1972.

Francouer, R.T. *Becoming a Sexual Person*. New York: John Wiley and Sons, 1982.

Friday, N. *My Secret Garden: Women's Sexual Fantasies*. New York: Pocket Books, 1973.

Hite, S. *The Hite Report*. New York: Warner, 1974.

"J." *The Sensuous Woman*. New York: Dell, 1969.

Kaplan, H. *The New Sex Therapy*. New York: Brunner/Mazel, 1974.

Katchadourian, H.A. & Lunde, D.T. *Fundamentals of Human Sexuality*. New York: Holt, Rinehart & Winston, 1972.

Ladas, Whipple, & Perry. *The "G" Spot*. New York: Holt, Rinehart & Winston.

Lowen, A. *Stress and Illness*. International Institute for Bioenergetic Analysis, 1980.

Masters, W.H. & Johnson, V. *Human Sexual Response*. Boston: Little, Brown, 1966.

————. *Human Sexual Inadequacy*. Boston: Little, Brown, 1970.

McCarthy, Barry. *Sexual Awareness, A Practical Approach*. San Francisco: Boyd & Fraser, Scrimshaw Press, 1975.

McCary, J.L. *Sexual Myths and Fallacies*. New York: Van Nostrand, 1971.

————. *Human Sexuality*. (second edition) New York: Van Nostrand, 1973.

Olds, Sally W. *The Eternal Garden: The Seasons of Our Sexuality*. New York: Times Books, 1985.

Reuben, D. *Everything You Always Wanted to Know About Sex, But Were Afraid to Ask*. New York: Bantam, 1969.

Rosenberg, Jack. *Total Orgasm*. New York: Random House.

Sarrel, Lorna and Sarrel, Phillip, M. *Sexual Turning Points: The Seven Stages of Adult Sexuality*. New York: Macmillan Publishing Company, 1984.

GENERAL

Bogin, Meg. *The Path to Pain Control*. Boston: Houghton Mifflin, 1982.

Brody, Jane. *Jane Brody's Nutrition Book*. New York: Bantam, 1981.

Burns, David. *Feeling Good: The New Mood Therapy*. New York: Signet, 1980.

Cousins, Norman. *Anatomy of an Illness*. New York: Bantam, 1979.

Fonda, Jane and McCarthy, Mignon. *Women Coming of Age*. New York: Simon and Schuster, 1984.

Gawain, Shakti Gawain. *Creative Visualization*. New York: Bantam, 1979.

Huttman, Barbara. *The Patient's Advocate: The Complete Handbook of Patient's Rights*. New York: Penguin, 1981.

Inlander, Charles and Weiner, Ed. *Take This Book to the Hospital with You*. Emmaus, PA: Rodale, 1985.

Kloss, Jethro. *Back to Eden: The Classic Guide to Herbal Medicine, Natural Foods, and Home Remedies*. Santa Barbara, CA: Lifeline, 1974.

Kushner, Harold S. *When Bad Things Happen to Good People*. New York: Schocken Books, 1981.

Lichtendorf, Susan. *Eve's Journey: The Physical Experience of Being Female*. New York: Putnam, 1982.

Matthews-Simonton, S. *The Healing Family: The Simonton Approach for Families Facing Illness*. New York: Bantam, 1984.

Porcino, Jane. *Growing Older, Getting Better: A Handbook for Women in the Second Half of Life*. Reading, MA: Addison-Wesley, 1983.

Shorr, Joseph. *Go See the Movie in Your Head*. New York: Popular Library, 1977.

Simonton, O.C., Matthews-Simonton, S. & Creighton, J. *Getting Well Again*. New York: Bantam, 1978.

Sobel, David S. & Ferguson, Tom. *The People's Book of Medical Tests*. New York: Summit, 1985.

Weinstein, Kate. *Endometriosis*. Reading, MA: Addison-Wesley, Forthcoming.

ARTICLES OF INTEREST

Beauchamp, Pedro & Held, Berel. "Estrogen Replacement Therapy." *Postgraduate Medicine* 75:7 (May 15, 1984).

Budoff, Penny. "Cyclic Estrogen–Progesterone Therapy." *American Medical Women's Association Journal* 39:1 (January/February, 1984).

Bush, Trudy, Cowan, Linda, Barrett-Conner, Elizabeth, and others. "Estrogen Use and All-Cause Mortality:" Preliminary Results from the Lipid Research Clinics Program Follow-Up Study. *JAMA* 249:7 (February 18, 1983).

Dicker, R., Scally, M., Greenspan, J. et al. "Hysterectomy Among Women of Reproductive Age: Trends in the United States, 1970-1978." *JAMA* 248:3 (July 16, 1982).

Hiatt, R., Bawol, R., Friedman, G., & Hoover, R. "Exogenous Estrogen and Breast Cancer After Bilateral Oophorectomy." *Cancer* 54 (1984).

Hughes, Jill. "Helplessness and Frustration: The Relatives' Dilemma." *Nursing Times* (June 9, 1982).

Kaltreider, N., Wallace, A., & Horowitz, M. "A Field Study of the Stress Response Syndrome": Young Women After Hysterectomy. *JAMA* 242:14 (October 5, 1979).

Keith, Carolyn. "Discussion Group for Posthysterectomy Patients." *Health and Social Work* (1980).

Krueger, J., Hassell, J., Goggins, D. et al. "Relationship Between Nurse Counseling and Sexual Adjustment after Hysterectomy." *Nursing Research* 28:3 (May/June, 1979).

MacMillan, Patricia. "Coming Home." *Nursing Times* (March 27, 1980).

Roeske, Nancy. "Quality of Life and Factors Affecting the Response to Hysterectomy." *Journal of Family Practice* 7:3 (1978).

Rowe, Dorothy. "Helping the Depressed Patient." *Nursing Times* (October 26, 1983).

Ruegsegger, P., Dambacher, M., Ruegsegger, M., and others. "Bone Loss in Premenopausal and Postmenopausal Women." *Journal of Bone and Joint Surgery* 66A:7 (September, 1984).

Sloan, Don. "The Emotional and Psychosexual Aspects of Hysterectomy." *The American Journal of Obstetrics and Gynecology* 131 (July 15, 1978).

JOURNALS PERTAINING TO GYNECOLOGICAL HEALTH

American Journal of Obstetrics & Gynecology
Biology of Reproduction
British Journal of Obstetrics & Gynecology
Endocrinology
Fertility & Sterility
Gynecologic & Obstetric Investigation
Gynecologic Oncology
Journal of Endocrinology
Obstetrics & Gynecology Survey

JOURNALS CONTAINING ARTICLES ON WOMEN'S HEALTH

Lancet
New England Journal of Medicine
Nurse Practitioner
Nursing Times
Women & Health

S O U R C E   N O T E S

1. Percentages were gathered from the National Center for Health Statistics, Hospital Discharge Survey (1983).
2. Adenomyosis—Fogel, Catherine & Woods, Nancy. *Health Care of Women—A Nursing Perspective.* St. Louis: Mosby, 1981.
3. PID. Fogel, Catherine & Woods, Nancy. *Health Care of Women—A Nursing Perspective.* St. Louis: Mosby, 1981.
4. Cervical cancer age groups—Romney, S., Gray, M.J., Little, A.B. and others, editors: *Gynecology and Obstetrics: The Health Care of Women.* New York: McGraw-Hill, 1975.
5. Cervical cancer and venereal disease—Disaia, P.J., Morrow, C.P., Townsend, D.E. *Synopsis of Gynecologic Oncology.* New York: John Wiley & Sons, 1975.
6. Ovarian cancer mortality—American Cancer Society. *The Facts and Figures.* New York: The Society, 1984.
7. Low grade malignancy—Romney, S. and others. *Gynecology and Obstetrics: The Health Care of Women.* New York: McGraw-Hill, 1975.
8. Percentages of abdominal hysterectomies—Barter, R. and others. *Controversy in Obstetrics and Gynecology.* Philadelphia: W. B. Saunders, 1974.
9. Hot flush—Rinehart, John & Schiff, Isaac. "Hormonal Imbalance; Hormonal Treatment." *Menopause Update* 1:2 (August, 1983): 13-16.
10. Biofeedback and flash/flush episodes—Unpublished personal survey of biofeedback therapists around the United States (1985).
11. Vitamin E and hot flashes—Seaman, Barbara & Seaman, Gideon. *Women and the Crisis in Sex Hormones.* New York: Bantam, 1977.
12. Ginseng and menopausal symptoms—Seaman, Barbara & Seaman, Gideon. *Women and the Crisis in Sex Hormones.* New York: Bantam, 1977.
13. Imagery and the mind-body connection—Unpublished personal conversation with Washington area psychiatrists currently involved in research with cancer patients and the use of imagery (March, 1985).
14. Kegel exercises and muscle tone—Perry, J.D. & Whipple, B. "Vaginal Myography." *Circumvaginal Musculature and Sexual Function.* Karger, 1982.
15. HRT and Migraines—Edelson, Richard. "Menstrual Migraine and Other Hormonal Aspects of Migraine." Unpublished paper (March, 1984).
16. Clonidine as used in controlling menopausal symptoms—Budoff, Penny. *No More Hot Flashes: And Other Good News.* New York: Warner, 1984.

I N D E X

Abdominal hysterectomy, 11, 36
Acceptance, and grief, 52-53
Accoutrements, for hospital stay, 32-33
Adenomyosis, 7-9
Admission procedures, and tests, hospital, 29-32
Alcohol, and osteoporosis, 67-68
American College of Obstetricians and Gynecologists, 19
Anaprox, 8
Anesthesia, risk, 38
Anger, and grief, 50-51
Assessment, of sexual self-esteem, 83-90
Atrophy, vaginal, and surgical menopause, 63-64
Authorization, for medical care and treatment, 43-44

Bargaining, and grief, 51
Barium enema, 30-31
Bear-down-and-relax exercise, 80
Bellergal, 73
Bilateral salpingo-oophorectomy, 11, 36
Biofeedback, and hot flash/flush, 60
Biopsy, endometrial, 11
Bladder, damage, 38
Blood count, complete (cbc), 30
Bloody type, cross and match, 30

Boston Women's Health Book Collective, 12
Bowel obstruction, 37

Caffeine, and osteoporosis, 67-68
Calcium
  in common foods, 73-75
  and osteoporosis, 67
Cancer, 9-11
Cervix, cancer of, 9-10
Chest X-ray, 30
Chlamydia, 9
Chocolate cysts, 6
Clonidine, 73
Communication, physician, 20-24
Compassion, physician, 24-25
Conization, 9
Consent forms, hospital, 46-48
Cortical tissue, bone, 65-66
Costs, physician and hospital, 29-30
Credentials, physician, 18-20

Danazol, 6, 7-8
D&C (dilatation and curettage), 11
Denial, and grief, 50
Depression
  checklist, 55-56
  and grief, 52-55
Diet, and recovery, 40
Disease, research on, 12-15

Vitamins
   and hot flash/flush, 60-61
   and osteoporosis, 67
   and vaginal atrophy, 63

Waletzky, Lucy, 110-11
Ware, Marsha, 67
Warning signs, osteoporosis, 66-67
Wound, separation, 38

Wanda Wigfall-Williams was born in Ochos Rios, Jamaica in 1953. She moved to Philadelphia in 1966 where she attended the Ancilla Domini Academy. Following her graduation, she enrolled in the honors program at Temple University, where she received her undergraduate degree in psychology. She continued her studies at the University of Pennsylvania where she earned a Master's Degree in the same subject.

Wanda Wigfall-Williams is now a clinical psychologist with vast experience in counseling women recovering from gynecological surgery. Her patient population includes domestic violence victims, child abuse victims, terminally ill children and adults, and rape victims.

Wigfall-Williams co-founded WOAR (Woman Organized Against Rape) in Philadelphia; has extensive involvement with the Hospice of Northern Virginia, where she serves on the Executive Committee of the Board of Directors, chairs the Volunteer Advisory Committee, and serves as a member of the Patient Care Committee. In addition, she serves on the Board of Directors of the Greater Washington, D.C. Chapter of the Endometriosis Association.

Ms. Wigfall-Williams resides in Virginia with her husband, David Gump, and their 12-year-old son, Chris.